GOD'S
DIET

GOD'S DIET

A Short and Simple Way
to Eat Naturally, Lose Weight,
and Live a Healthier Life

DOROTHY GAULT-McNEMEE, M.D.

Harmony Books
New York

Copyright © 1995, 1996, 1999 Dorothy Gault-McNemee, M.D.

Published by Harmony Books, 201 East 50th Street, New York, New York 10022. Member of the Crown Publishing Group.

Random House, Inc. New York, Toronto, London, Sydney, Auckland
www.randomhouse.com

HARMONY BOOKS is a registered trademark and Harmony Books colophon is a trademark of Random House, Inc.

Originally published in two previous editions by the author in 1995 and 1996.

Printed in the United States of America

Design by Meryl Sussman Levavi/Digitext

Library of Congress Cataloging-in-Publication Data
Gault-McNemee, Dorothy.
    God's diet : a short and simple way to eat naturally, lose weight, and live a healthier life / Dorothy Gault-McNemee.
        p.   cm.
    1. Reducing diets. 2. Weight loss. I. Title.
    RM222.G38   1999
    613.2'5—dc21   99-33057
                                                              CIP

ISBN 0-609-60517-8

10 9 8 7 6 5 4 3 2 1

Revised and updated edition

To all of the chubs of the world.

To my mother,
Alice Gault,
who laid the groundwork for intelligent eating.

To my husband,
Richard McNemee,
who has made my life complete.

To my Heavenly Father, who loves me and taught
me the following principles so I could share them
with you.

ACKNOWLEDGMENTS

❧

I would like to thank all of my patients who have helped in the development of my diet program. We have all learned together. I would also like to thank them for giving up their blood to prove that their cholesterol and triglycerides really do go down with this way of eating.

I would like to gratefully acknowledge the following people for the work they did editing the first edition of this book: my mother, Alice Gault; my sister, Florence Schetgen; her colleague, Gail Kushen; my husband, Richard McNemee; and our Clinic Manager and friend, Annalee Johnson. Thanks also to Shaye Areheart for the careful editing and great suggestions for this edition and to Mary Ann Naples for all of her confidence and support.

I would especially like to thank Laurie Beth Jones, author of *Jesus, CEO; The Path; Jesus in Blue Jeans;* and *Grow Something Besides Old,* for getting sick and coming to the clinic and then inquiring about my book; for taking the time to read it and then sending it to her agent. Laurie and I both truly believe that God led her to me so this book would be able to reach everyone. May God also lead you to healthier eating and living.

CONTENTS

✿

GOD'S DIET

IF GOD DIDN'T MAKE IT, DON'T EAT IT

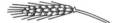

Now, if you want to spend good money for this book, go ahead. But if you understand the chapter title, spend your money for something else.

I've made this book short for two reasons: because the concept is so easy it doesn't need a long book and because I want you to read the book and change your life.

❊

Since I was thirteen years old, I have bounced from one diet to another, spending far too much money on diet books and fad diets. I finally just gave up. The research was telling me that I was born with my fat genes and it really wasn't my fault that I was overweight. I was finally fed up (no pun intended) and decided to eat whatever I wanted and forget about my weight. (That little decision was good for another 15 pounds!!!)

I am sure it comes as no surprise that even as I was eating

with no restrictions, I still wasn't happy. So, over the next year I spent a lot of time thinking about the diets that worked, and those that didn't. I knew deep in my heart that pasta and six slices of bread a day wasn't good for me, no matter what the nutritionists were telling my diabetic patients. I knew that cutting out all of the fat in my diet would help me lose weight; however, I also knew that my body wouldn't have the building blocks it needed to make hormones, that my skin would get dry and my hair would get brittle if I didn't have fat. I also knew that I needed fat in my diet to feel full as well as to absorb the fat-soluble vitamins.

I felt I no longer had the time nor the inclination to count calories, fat grams or carbos. I didn't want to weigh 2 ounces of this or 4 ounces of that. I had always had a hard time remembering how many bread exchanges, fat exchanges, vegetable and fruit exchanges are deemed "healthy." I couldn't remember which diet was better—the Asian or Mediterranean or American Pyramid plan. I couldn't remember what was on any of their meal plans. And even if I could remember, I certainly threw out all of my knowledge the moment I stepped into a restaurant.

Then one day the front page of the newspaper said that "XYZ" was good for you while the folks on TV said that it was bad for you. All on the same day! That was when I threw up my arms and said, "If God didn't make it, don't eat it."

I realized that what I really wanted was to be healthy and trim. Logic said that I needed to go back to basics—and when I say basics, I mean back to 10,000-to-15,000-years-ago-type basics. I've often told my patients that we chubs come from good stock. We are the survivors. We are the ones whose ancestors stored body fat efficiently for the lean years. So, since we obviously hadn't evolved to be able to eat whatever and whenever, we were obviously going to have to go back to basics. We were going to have to go back and eat the way we did when we first appeared on the earth thousands of years ago—and the way we had eaten until the last hundred years. We were going to have to be logical.

If God made us and made all of the animals, fruits, and vegetables, then that must be what we were intended to eat. Obviously, we've been around a pretty long time. So, I decided to disregard all of the information about low-fat diets and pasta being good for you. I decided that weighing food and counting calories, or fat, or carbohydrates or anything else just didn't make sense. I didn't need to add more work to my life.

Knowing that there really had to be a healthy way to eat good food and feel satisfied, I developed God's Diet. Actually, this easy, effective way of eating was there all of the time; I just read the signposts. It is really so simple. I call it God's Diet because a name like "All Natural" implies that anything that isn't a manmade chemical would be okay. It is those very products that are often loaded with sugar and flour, and *that* is *not okay.* Once we begin to process food, we tend to take away all its good, nutritional qualities and leave all that is bad. And for good measure, we'll add some sugar or corn syrup!

Think of it this way: if it wasn't around 10,000 to 15,000 years ago, you probably shouldn't be eating it. I can't imagine Adam and Eve throwing together a little pasta with Alfredo sauce (one of my personal favorites). I bet they didn't bake nicely crusted bread. They didn't have luscious donuts, or birthday cake with ice cream. They didn't make enchiladas or gorditas. They either killed it, picked it, or dug it up. If it was good enough for them, why not try it ourselves? It certainly seemed logical. (If I am nothing else, I am logical.) Of course, we also know that our ancient ancestors often died in their twenties and thirties. But they didn't die of heart attacks and clogged arteries or diabetes and obesity. Heck, they probably didn't have a word like *fat* in their vocabulary. They died because they were sick or wounded and couldn't go out and kill, gather, or pick. They died of deprivation and infections.

So, why not buy what we need and eat just what God provided for us? He certainly didn't provide us with all of the lovely but harmful goodies that have become so much a part of our lives.

Now, I can't imagine that there were pies, cakes, cookies, or candy around 10,000 years ago. But then, that one is easy—even I haven't found a diet that encourages any of that. When you start getting into bread, tortillas, and pasta you probably think you are *okay*. I contend that for us chubs, those things are *not okay*. I believe that sugar and flour are our enemies. I also think they are addictive. For example, have you ever been able to eat only one donut? Not I. I always had the second one and really wanted to finish off the rest of the box. Only guilt and a small amount of self-control kept me from doing that.

So, just what did God create? Following is a list of what He made and one of what He didn't. I have also added a swing list—foods that are not okay but are not bad enough to never eat again.

Obviously, the lists are not all-inclusive, but I think you will get the idea. As you read the lists, see if you don't grasp the simple logic in them.

FOODS YOU CAN HAVE

abalone
alfalfa sprouts
apples
apricots
artichokes
arugula
asparagus
avocado
bacon
bamboo shoots
bananas
beans (all kinds)
beef
beets
blackberries
blueberries
broccoli
Brussels sprouts
butter
cabbage
cantaloupe
carrots
cauliflower
celery
chard or Swiss chard
cherries
chicken
chives
cilantro
clams

corn
cracked wheat
cranberries
cucumbers
daikon
dates
dill pickles
duck
eggplant
eggs
endive
figs
fish (any kind)
garlic
ginger root
goat
grapefruit
grapes
green peppers
green beans
greens (beet, collard, dandelion, mustard, turnip)
guava
ham
homemade salsa
honey
jalapeños
jicama
kale
kelp
kiwi fruit
kohlrabi
kumquats
lamb
leeks

lemons
lettuce (any variety)
limes
litchis
liver (I bet that one makes you happy)
lobster
lotus root
mamey (a tropical fruit)
mangos
melons
milk
mushrooms
mustard
nectarines
nuts
oatmeal
okra
oil (olive or canola are best)
olives
onions
oranges
oysters
papaya
parsley
parsnips
passion fruit
peas
peaches
pears
pepper (black)
peppers (chili)
peppers (red and green)
persimmon
pheasant

picante sauce	scallions
Pico de Gallo	scallops
pineapple	seaweed
plums	shallots
pomegranate	shrimp
pork	soy
potatoes (sweet, Idaho, etc.)	spices
	spinach
prickly pear	squab
prunes	squash
pumpkin	strawberries
quail	string beans
quince	tangerines
rabbit	tomatoes
radishes	turkey
raisins	turnips
raspberries	venison
rhubarb	vinegar
rice (brown, long cooking)	water chestnuts
rutabaga	watercress
salmon	watermelon
salt	whole wheat

This list does not include all of the wonderful foods that God made. If you aren't sure about an item, ask yourself "Did God make it?" Remember, God made every fruit, every vegetable, and every meat, fish, and fowl. If you can't pick it from a tree or vine, or pull it out of the ground or kill it, then you probably shouldn't eat it.

If your friends and family quip and say that God made the sugar and the wheat that goes into your cake, then you can justify any food. And once you make those concessions, you'll be hooked on sugar and flour again and will start to gain weight instead of lose it. All that sugar and flour and processed food is the cause of the trouble for all of us chubs. The things you can't have follow.

FOODS YOU CAN'T HAVE

ALCOHOL (including wine and beer)
bagels
BREAD
cake
candy
catsup
cereals (except for those on the swing list)
cold cuts (most of them)
cookies
corn syrup
cornstarch
crackers
flour
marshmallows
PASTA
pie
pita bread
salad dressing (except for those on the swing list)
sugar*
sweet pickles
tortillas (flour)
yogurt (most of them)

Unfortunately, while labeling is now mandatory for all of our foods, the labelers have become very creative in hiding the truth of what is in their products. Packaging that says "sugar free—sweetened with fructose" is criminal. For those who don't know that fructose is still sugar, this particular food item becomes poison for diabetics and for other people who are trying to limit the amount of sugar in their diets.

The latest trick is to sell "dehydrated cane juice." (Sugar by

---

*Sugar includes any of the added sugars, such as fructose, glucose, sucrose, maltose, lactose, dextrose, and galactose.

any other name is still *sugar.*) Heck, it is enough to make one paranoid!

Another ingredient found in some food, modified food starch, is a poison for us. If you find it on your packaged food ingredient label, don't eat that product. It has no nutritional value and acts just like sugar to make us crave more.

Beware of any canned or packaged food. Read the ingredients, not the amount of calories, fat, protein, and carbohydrates. Why the ingredients and not the number of grams or calories of each item? Because grams of sugar or carbohydrate are not always equal. For example, the natural sugar in an apple is fructose. If you have an apple in one hand and fructose from another apple in the other hand, we've been told that those two fructoses are equal. They are *not* equal. The fructose in the apple has to be eaten and then digested as well. The body will not be 100 percent efficient in getting all those grams of fructose out of the apple. We will use calories to do the digesting. Then the apple will act like the fiber it is to help with good bowel movements. That processed fructose, on the other hand, can be easily and totally digested and utilized and won't act as fiber, either. Minimal calories will be utilized to process the "processed" fructose. So you see, it is the sugar that is *added* to our food that is so bad, rather than the sugar that is in the food naturally.

That is not to say that having unlimited naturally packaged sugar is okay. For example, eleven bananas a day is not intelligent eating. You can eat only fruit all day and not lose weight. If our kids are drinking orange juice all day instead of water, they will get fat.

Beware of any food product that says "low fat" or "all natural." Those are often the worst for added sugar, corn syrup, or cornstarch. Marketing people have convinced us that "low fat" and "all natural" products are good for us. However, when they take out some or all of the fat or the preservatives, they often add sugar or cornstarch.

If you think that you are going to suffer on God's Diet, then you aren't reading carefully enough. How could anyone feel deprived while eating a steak and a baked potato with butter? As you start to read the labels of the foods you've been eating, you'll get longer and longer lists of things you shouldn't have been eating. But you will also get longer and longer lists of food you can eat and haven't been. If you don't understand the words on a package label, then don't eat it. You must start to think of any food that is packaged as being potentially contaminated with sugar, flour, corn syrup, and cornstarch. The package the manufacturer provides must convince you otherwise.

Your new motto is: IF GOD DIDN'T MAKE IT, DON'T EAT IT.

Now, there are a few foods I am sure you noticed weren't on either list. These foods I am going to put on a swing list. These are the foods that are not recommended when you are being a purist. These are foods that should be used rarely. We'll talk a little more about why these foods are not good, but not totally bad either.

SWING LIST

artificial sweeteners
cheese
corn tortillas
cottage cheese
cream cheese
Grape-Nuts
honey
Jell-O (diet)
Marie's Blue Cheese Dressing
Paul Newman's Vinegar and Oil Dressing
popcorn
Shredded Wheat
soda pop (no more than one a day)
sour cream (pure)
tea and coffee (no more than two a day, and
    decaf would be better)
yogurt (some)

Cheese, cream cheese, cottage cheese, and sour cream should be used sparingly. While they are nutritionally good, when man processed them, he compacted those calories so we don't have to work hard to extract the calories. Do not use these as a main meal, but rather as a garnish.

Yogurt is like cheese in that it is nutritionally sound but is really dense with calories. However, the bigger problem with yogurt is that practically all of them have had sugar added to them. When you buy yogurt be very careful when reading the label. (When I was in medical school I went on an 800-calorie-a-day diet of just yogurt—and didn't lose weight.) It is not only the calories we eat, but where those calories are coming from that dictates how much weight we lose. That is why counting calories or counting anything else just doesn't work.

While Marie's Blue Cheese Dressing, Paul Newman's Vinegar and Oil Dressing, and other dressings may be LEGAL, use them sparingly. They are also jam-packed with concentrated calories.

So what do I mean when I talk about LEGAL?

LEGAL means that God made it or that when it was being processed by man, at least man didn't add sugar, flour, corn syrup, or cornstarch. Example: God made strawberries.

ILLEGAL (or sinful) means that it wasn't made by God or that sugar, flour, corn syrup, or cornstarch has been added to it. Example: Man packaged the strawberries but added sugar before freezing the strawberries.

That is why this way of eating is really so easy. If you go to a restaurant and you are trying to decide what to order, just ask yourself if God made it. This way of eating is just plain old logical.

Honey is pure sugar. Yes, God made it. If you want it in unlimited quantities, then you had better be prepared to go out and gather your own, not pour it from a bottle. Think about it. You are an ancient ancestor, wearing your animal skins, and you come across a beehive. You take a big stick and knock the hive down. Assuming you survive the hundreds of bee stings, you will treat the honey as if it were really precious. When you put that honey on your cereal or in your tea, is that the way you are thinking about it—that it is so precious that it was worth dying for? If it isn't worth dying for, then I suggest that you cut way back on the honey.

Now let's talk about coffee and tea. No calories, right? Should be able to have in unlimited quantities, especially if you don't add anything to it. That was the old thinking when you and I used to count calories. We know more now. We know that caffeine stimulates the pancreas to produce insulin, which grabs onto the glucose running around in our blood and deposits it onto our hips as fat. So why would we want to do that? Doesn't compute. While most people think they can't survive without the caffeine, we really can. Yes, you can have one or two cups of caffeine a day if you feel you must, but you will lose weight faster and actually feel better if you get that caffeine way down—to zero if you're really motivated.

As for soda, even when it is sugar free and caffeine free, you should limit it to a maximum of one a day—again, to rarely or not at all is the best. When we have too much artificial sweetener, it seems to really slow down the weight loss.

As for those artificial sweeteners, if you can eliminate them it would be wonderful. If you can only stick with this way of eating because you can have some artificial sweeteners, then have them—but be stingy with them. God didn't make them.

Tortillas are on the swing list, as is popcorn. I often hear about tortillas being just corn, so why can't the person have it. After all, they can have plain corn. Good question. (Obviously, flour tortillas will never pass your lips again.) Let's go back to plain corn before moving onto the corn tortillas and the popcorn, since I've told you that you can have plain kernel corn. When you have plain corn or corn on the cob, and then you check your stool (poop) the next day, what do you see? Corn! It seems that we human beings just aren't all that efficient when it comes to digesting corn. However, when we pop the corn, we open up the outer coating, which now makes the corn easily digestible and fattening. The same thing happens when we make masa for corn tortillas. We dissolve that outer coating off of the corn (in lye, no less) and now the masa is made into an easily digestible and fattening tortilla. That is why corn is used to fatten up cattle. They chew their cud and have four stomachs. They are able to digest the corn without having to make it into popcorn or masa first. When we make it into popcorn or masa, then the corn is as fattening for us as it is for the cattle.

Diet Jell-O is all processed food. However, it opens up a lot of variety into our meals, so you can have *some*. Once again, it should not be a staple in your daily eating because it can slow down the weight loss.

There will always be more items that haven't been listed. Remember to use common sense and logic if you don't know about an item. Could you pluck it off a tree or vine? Could you kill it? Could you dig it out of the ground? If the answer is no to all of those questions, then you probably shouldn't eat it (unless it is eggs or milk, which don't fit into any of those categories; but then you already know about eggs and milk—you can have them). Speaking of common sense and logic, while God made some poisonous plants and poisonous fish, He didn't mean for us to eat them.

CHAPTER 2

WE'RE KILLING OURSELVES!

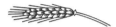

Now I'd like to share with you a little of what the press has reported. An article printed in the *El Paso Times* on January 17, 1996, from the Gannett News Service quoted several authorities who said the following:

Americans eat more, pass on exercise.

Despite all the badgering to eat better and exercise regularly, Americans still aren't, a new federal report shows.

People are eating more calories than they did a few years ago. And even though they're eating lower fat food, they're eating more fat simply because they're eating more. They're not eating their dark green or yellow vegetables.

On top of that, many aren't exercising vigorously.

Participants reported weighing an average of 11–12 pounds more in 1994 than they did in the late 70s.

The Centers for Disease Control and Prevention announced in November 1998 that the high-fat, high-carbohydrate snacks that have made our teenagers obese have also triggered Type 2 diabetes.[1] While a formal study has not yet been done, it appears that the number of these cases has *tripled* in the past five years. Here are some statistics I have picked up from various sources:

> Americans spend about $33 billion a year trying to shed pounds.[2]

> One type of cancer of the esophagus has increased more than 350 percent among white men in the past twenty years, and the researchers say the reasons may include smoking and an increase in obesity.[3]

> As for dietary cholesterol, studies demonstrate little effect of reducing intake of foods containing cholesterol in most adults and no effect in a sizable subset of otherwise healthy subjects.[4]

> Obese women or those who have gained more than 44 pounds since they were 18 years old are about two and a half times more likely to suffer ischemic and total stroke than lean women who have not gained weight.[5]

> Table sugar may shorten life span and increase aging. Researchers theorize that excessive sugar ultimately generates free radical chemicals that mess up proteins and accelerate the aging process, causing disease and premature death.[6]

Some statistics from the *Journal of the American Medical Association* indicate that one in every three adults is overweight; obesity accounts for more than $68 billion per year in excess health-care costs and loss of income. We spend over $30 billion per year on diet foods, diet products, and diet programs; and physicians are more likely to treat the conditions exacerbated by weight gain (such as diabetes, cardiovascular disease, hypertension) than to treat obesity itself.[7]

Okay, now let's take a look at all of this with our "newly discovered" God's Diet. We are eating more calories because when fat is taken out of a food, sugar or corn syrup is often added to get back some of the taste. When we eat sugar and corn syrup (both of which are non-fat, by the way), we are getting addicted to it. Once we are addicted, we have begun our downward spiral of eating more and more sugar and calories.

We are being told we are getting fatter. Of course we are getting fatter. How could we be getting skinnier when we are eating more total calories?

We aren't getting vigorous exercise either. Did you ever carry around a 12-pound backpack while jogging, let alone a 50- or 100-pound backpack? When we are fat, it is too hard to exercise. And haven't we all heard that you shouldn't start an exercise program without seeing your doctor first, or you might have a heart attack? So then we end up becoming discouraged about exercising vigorously when we are more than a few pounds overweight. We certainly don't want to go to the doctor and be told we're *fat;* we already know that! So we end up not exercising.

We are told to eat a balanced diet. By whose standards? What is a balanced diet?

What about a diabetic diet? Why are all these bread exchanges good for us? Who do you know who ever stayed on any of those exchange diets? Who can keep it all straight? One study says we shouldn't drink alcohol, the next study says a glass of wine per day is good (though not if you're an alcoholic). Fat is bad. Eggs were bad but now they are okay again. Pasta is good. (Now give me a break. How did we ever believe that one? Pasta is nothing more than refined flour made into strips or squares.) We've equated pasta with good food; therefore we thought we were dieting when we ate it. We get so many mixed messages and become so confused, we end up giving up—and getting fatter and fatter. And why shouldn't we be confused. It certainly seems that our doctors and nutritionists are confused. I was as confused as everyone else was until I literally gave up. That was the start of God's Diet: going back to basics and logic.

With God's Diet, you will eat very well. You won't have to worry anymore. You won't have to count or weigh food anymore. You don't have to keep a meal log. You don't have to figure out exchanges. You hardly have to think anymore. If God didn't make it, don't eat it. Period. Punto. Fini.

I read an article that states that scientists have located a genetic mutation in mice that accounted for some forms of obesity. However, I was wondering if there could also be a mutated gene that accounts for skinny? Let's face it, we all know people who can eat anything—even all those cakes, cookies, and desserts that you and I shouldn't eat. Well, I certainly don't have any "skinny" genes, and while I may have some fat genes, I believe our biggest problem is eating all those high-sugar fast foods. We are still the same as we were 10,000 years ago. Therefore, we still should eat the food that God made, not that man made. So, you think that isn't fair? Maybe not, but we can still have steak and a baked potato and that sure isn't suffering.

We've all heard that we have our own "set point," and that our bodies have a weight that it tries to maintain. I believe that. However, I think that our set point is lower than most of us chubs decided it probably was. I think we have been so misguided as to what we should eat, that we couldn't possibly get down to our "true" set point as long as we eat foods that are bad for us.

To show you how really poor the public school dieticians' example of a "good diet" is, I am going to list a random day of school menus from around El Paso, Texas, as published in the *El Paso Times* on March 7, 1999.[8] If our schools are a place of learning, then we should be teaching intelligent eating. At this rate, the next generation will be dead of fat, hypertension, and diabetes before they reach forty.

ANTHONY:
> Breakfast: WAFFLES, sausage or oatmeal, TOAST, apple slices
>
> Lunch: HOT DOGS, PORK AND BEANS, orange in wedges

CANUTILLO:
> Breakfast: BREAKFAST BURRITO, salsa
>
> Lunch: RIB-B-QUE ON A BUN, lettuce, tomato, PICKLE, TATER TOTS, KETCHUP

EL PASO:
> Breakfast: Juice, CINNAMON TOAST, TEXAS TOAST AND CEREAL
>
> Lunch: Taco salad or baked GLAZED ham, CANDIED SWEET POTATOES, AU GRATIN POTATOES, WHOLE WHEAT ROLL, fruit

FABENS:
> Breakfast: Hash browns, scrambled egg with ham, TOAST AND CEREAL
>
> Lunch: Chicken patty, CREAM GRAVY, mashed potatoes, veggies, ROLLS, apple

GADSDEN:
> Breakfast: COLD CEREAL WITH GRAHAM CRACKERS OR FRUIT TOASTIE, fruit juice
>
> Lunch: Chicken stir fry, oriental vegetables, ROLL, STEAMED RICE (WHITE), PORK AND BEANS, chilled fruit

SAN ELIZARIO:
> Breakfast: CEREAL, TOAST or EGG BURRITO, fresh fruit
>
> Lunch: Chicken patty, CREAM GRAVY, mashed potatoes, veggies, ROLLS, apple

SOCORRO:
> Breakfast: DRY CEREAL, TOAST, juice or PANCAKES WITH SYRUP, sausage patty

Lunch: Beef patty smothered with chili con queso, half
baked potato, WHEAT ROLL, orange wedges

TORNILLO:

Breakfast: Chorizo and potato BURRITO
Lunch: Chicken patty, mashed potatoes, veggies, ROLLS

YSLETA:

Breakfast: Spanish omelet with FLOUR TORTILLAS
Lunch: SPAGHETTI with meat sauce, tossed salad, pear
halves, GARLIC ROLL

I capitalized the bad food, so if you plowed through all of that,
you can see that this way of eating is wrong. How can we
allow our children to eat so much sugar and flour? No wonder
everyone is getting fatter when we teach good nutrition with
this kind of menu.

After this heavy sugar load for breakfast and then lunch,
the "normal" kids will have a dip in their blood sugar levels
and have a hard time staying awake for class. The kids who are
hyperactive and sensitive to sugar will be bouncing off the
walls after they eat. (At least they might keep the others awake.)
It is no wonder that we have so much ADHD (Attention Deficit
Hyperactivity Disorder) when we are literally throwing sugar at
them. (No, I am not saying that there is no such thing as
ADHD; I do believe we are over-diagnosing this condition. Too
many people think these kids only need Ritalin to calm down.
I think a large number of them also need healthy diets, and
with better eating they might need less medication.)

Here's another interesting tidbit. Some recent studies con-
ducted by Roger McDonald and his colleagues at the University
of California at Davis show that when rats were allowed to eat
all of the sugar they wanted, they aged and died prematurely
(see note 6). When the rats were allowed only 60 percent as
much table sugar, they lived about 35 percent longer than
those who ate sugar freely. Merely restricting calories can
increase survival, but that was not the whole story. Rats who

ate equal calories in starchy carbohydrates also lived about 20 percent longer than heavy sugar eaters.

I know we aren't rats, but it's obvious that rats haven't mutated, either. They can't eat all this refined sugar without detriment any more than we can. And with their life spans being shorter than ours, they certainly would have been able to mutate faster than we can.

We know that certain foods can actually help us. Certain foods can boost your mood. Turkey, for instance, is rich in an amino acid called tyrosine, which boosts levels of the brain chemicals dopamine and norepinephrine, and this, in turn, improves motivation and reaction time. Tuna and chicken also have lots of tyrosine.

Iron is needed to keep the body's cells fueled with oxygen and, thus, energized. Therefore, complete avoidance of red meat may do more harm than good. People on low-cholesterol diets may experience iron deficiencies that make them feel tired and blue. A 1992 study at Illinois State University, reported in *Reader's Digest* in February 1996, discovered that when people ate as little as 3 ounces of beef per day, they absorbed 50 percent more iron than those on a vegetarian diet.[9] So if you are a vegetarian, be sure you are taking an iron supplement. If you don't eat beef anymore, maybe you should reconsider why you don't. If you gave it up for your health, you may be causing more harm than good.

Mild dehydration is another common, but overlooked, cause of fatigue. When the body dehydrates, blood flow to the organs decreases, and the body slows down. Drinking enough water each day can prevent you from feeling lethargic. But don't rely on thirst as an indicator. Most adults should drink eight to ten 8-ounce glasses of water per day. Caffeinated soft drinks and coffee are no substitute. In fact, they actually act as diuretics and may increase dehydration and subsequent fatigue.

How many of us talk about all of the water we're carrying (especially when we females are PMSing) and hold back on our water intake thinking it will help the bloating? That turns out to be absolutely the worst thing we can do because water deprivation leads to mild dehydration and then we feel really bad. To feel better we turn to chocolate and sugar for a mental and physical boost, which in fact just increases the bloating. Instead we need to get rid of the sugar and increase our water intake, especially if suffering from PMS. Increasing water and eliminating sugar, flour, corn syrup, and cornstarch will decrease the water retention and increase energy levels.

Magnesium deficiency and stress are linked so closely that some doctors and dieticians advise people who lead hectic lives to add magnesium-rich foods to their diets. Bananas, nuts, beans, and leafy vegetables have lots of magnesium. If you juggle a hectic schedule, the problem is worse: stress hormones, which flood the body during times of tension, drain magnesium from cells, resulting in lower resistance to colds and other viruses and causing a tired feeling. Researchers have also found that increased magnesium intake results in less anxiety and better sleep (*Reader's Digest,* February 1996).

Even a small deficiency in vitamin C—a key ingredient for boosting levels of energizing norepinephrine—can leave you feeling irritable and blue. A lack of foods rich in vitamin C also inhibits your body's ability to absorb the iron it needs to fight fatigue. Another study found that diets containing vitamin C in a dose of 150 milligrams—roughly the amount in two oranges—resulted in a reduction of nervousness, crankiness, and depression.

Brazil nuts are loaded with selenium, a trace mineral that some research has linked to upbeat moods. A 1991 study at the University of Wales, Swansea, gave 100 micrograms of selenium per person per day. (This is the equivalent of one or two Brazil nuts). Those eating the nuts reported a great sense of happiness, more energy, and a reduction in anxiety compared to participants given a placebo. Other good sources of selenium include seafood and beef.

The January 8, 1996 issue of *U.S. News and World Report*

included an article entitled "Are You Too Fat?" It had distress-
ing information that a "third of Americans are overweight to
the point of obesity, up from a fourth in the 70s. And by
encouraging problems like heart disease and diabetes, obesity
thins the population by some 300,000 a year."

JAMA reported about women who had "put on 20 to 40
pounds since age 18 and matched them against women who
had held their weight. The gainers were two and a half times
more likely to die of coronary heart disease. Americans, it
seems, are replacing fat with seconds and thirds of everything
else." See note 5.

Doctors, dieticians, and all sorts of health gurus tell us to
lose weight and to exercise. How often have we chubs heard,
"Just eat less." "If you really wanted to lose weight, you
would." "Eat less of everything." (What? Less cake? I maintain,
no cake.) We are told pasta is good, so we eat lots of it. If it's
good, it must be a diet food and we can eat all we want of diet
food, right? Wrong. We need to go back to being logical. Pasta
was not in the Garden of Eden. It is not good for us. It makes
us fat and bloated. Even a little pasta keeps the weight on and
destroys our ability to lose weight. Unless you absolutely have
to eat someone's homemade pasta meal, avoid it like the
plague. They both can kill you.

I don't know about you, but I am tired of feeling deprived.
I don't want to weigh food before I eat it. I don't want to count
anything. I don't want to have to remember if I am supposed to
eat protein before carbohydrates or vice versa. It isn't that I am
lazy, I just have more important things to think about. That's
what's so nice about God's Diet; it is just logical. You are never
hungry. You can't feel deprived. You have the rules on how to
eat and they are simple: just eat the things that God made.

❦

One of my more eccentric patients has gone on my diet just to
prove me "crazy." She has high cholesterol and triglycerides.

She has been denying herself anything with cholesterol in it for eight years. She has taken lipid-lowering medicines to control her lipids even further. We had to stop those because it was affecting her liver. When I suggested she try God's Diet, she became quite indignant. When she finally decided to try it, she went to the other extreme. She couldn't wait to go out and buy steak and Brie cheese and every other fat-laden food she could think of.

As I explained to her, that is not what I am preaching. I am preaching a *balanced* diet. That does not mean eating unlimited amounts of fats, proteins, fruits, and starchy vegetables. I am telling people to have the food God made and to eat intelligently. Steak three times a day is not good, nor is eating only apples all day. This is not a crash diet nor a "cleansing" diet nor a lose-ten-pounds-in-a-week diet. This is a balanced diet that is *for life*. This is a diet that you can live with and one that will help you live longer. *This is a logical way to eat.* If you want food groups, let's talk about meat, fish and fowl, fruits and vegetables, and milk and milk products and grains. Let's not muddy the issue by overlooking all of those hidden sugars and flours that man has put into, poured over, and hidden under the good foods that God made. Remember, despite all of our medical advances, it seems that what we are eating is indeed killing us.

As I tell my patients, there is the letter of the law and the spirit of the law. Just because something is legal doesn't mean you overdo it. For example, dried fruit is okay. But don't eat twenty dried apricots per day. Would you eat ten fresh apricots in a day? If you would, then eat the fresh ones; they're better for you. Have the dried ones occasionally. When the fruit is dried, its natural sugar content becomes very concentrated and the dried fruit isn't as filling as the fresh is, so we end up eating more of the dried fruit.

How is it then, you ask, that we were able to have cake and candy and pie when we were younger? Well, first and foremost, when we were kids we were a lot more active than the kids of today. Now kids sit in front of their TVs, VCRs, and computers. When I was a kid, we didn't have a TV until I was seven and even then, Mom and Dad were smart enough to limit our TV time. The rest of the time was spent playing and expending energy or doing homework. Of course, as kids we also burned off the calories a lot quicker. But, I maintain there is a third reason. When I was growing up we never thought about having desserts every day. We didn't have access to donuts on a daily basis or even every weekend. When we had candy, it was because Mom made fudge. We certainly weren't allowed to squander our money on a candy bar. If we had pie, it was because we were having company. If we had cake it was because it was someone's birthday. Now we have snack foods any time, anywhere. We are always busy and on the run living hectic lives. When we run into a convenience store, snack foods loaded with sugar, flour, and fat are within reach of the cash register. We seldom have the option of buying an apple or an orange. No wonder we get fat. We go out to eat more than ever before. Rolls are always served and we usually top dinner off with a dessert. We'd be better off doing what the French do: finish the meal with cheese and fruit.

※

I've included a copy of the "U.S. Department of Agriculture's Food Guide Pyramid" because I believe it is incorrect (see table on page 36). It contains bad advice and is out of date. Just look at it. For us chubs, we've been very good about getting in our six to eleven servings of bread, cereal, rice, and pasta each day (as listed on the Food Guide Pyramid). If we kept it to the cereals without the sugar and non-processed rice, we'd be in better shape. The trouble is that food manufacturers have stripped away so much of the good stuff and then added sugar (that is, empty calories).

To take our minds off the sugar and calories and to make us think the food is good for us, they "fortify" it with vitamins

THE FOOD GUIDE PYRAMID

A GUIDE TO DAILY FOOD CHOICES

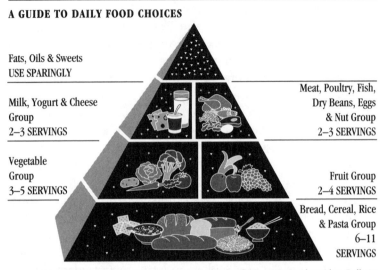

Fats, Oils & Sweets
USE SPARINGLY

Milk, Yogurt & Cheese
Group
2–3 SERVINGS

Meat, Poultry, Fish,
Dry Beans, Eggs
& Nut Group
2–3 SERVINGS

Vegetable
Group
3–5 SERVINGS

Fruit Group
2–4 SERVINGS

Bread, Cereal, Rice
& Pasta Group
6–11
SERVINGS

SOURCE: Reproduced from the U.S. Department of Agriculture Home and Garden Bulletin Number 252.

and minerals. If they had just left it alone in the first place, then the foods wouldn't need to be fortified.

I've also included the "Asian Pyramid" and the "Mediterranean Pyramid." It is suggested by some nutritional experts that we eat a few days like the Asians, a few days like the Mediterraneans, and one day like Americans, because the Asians and Mediterraneans aren't dying of diabetes and high blood pressure and other obesity-induced illnesses as young as we Americans are dying.

I don't know about you, but trying to remember how much of which pyramid on which day becomes so confusing that I'd just throw up my hands and eat whatever. And there are so many different messages. Recently, I heard that fruits were bad for you. Can you imagine? Anyway, has it occurred to anyone that the Asians and Mediterraneans are healthier because they don't eat all of the processed sugar and flour that we eat? Rather than try to keep some pyramid in your mind, you just need to remember that the more basic, the more

THE ASIAN PYRAMID

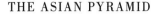

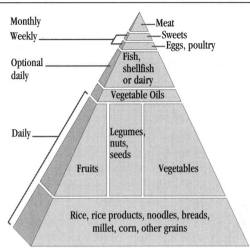

SOURCE: Copyright, January 8, 1996, U.S. News & World Report. Visit us at our Web site at www.usnews.com for additional information.

THE MEDITERRANEAN PYRAMID

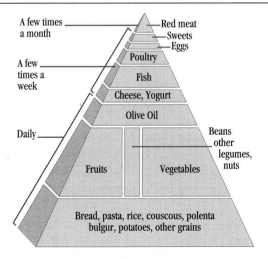

SOURCE: Copyright, January 8, 1996, U.S. News & World Report. Visit us at our Web site at www.usnews.com for additional information.

natural, the better. We have overwhelmed our senses and thus our bodies with the "good stuff." We are killing ourselves with the "good stuff."

You know, there wasn't a cigarette that I ever met that I didn't like. I gave up smoking anyway, because it wasn't good for me. And while I liked to smoke, it certainly wasn't worth dying for. The same for donuts—I never met one of those I didn't like either—but, again, it was not worth dying for. I believe that most of us chubs do want to be thinner, but we all certainly want to be healthier.

As for will power, we chubs have lots more will power than those "skinnies" we talked about. Who among them would ever have had the will power to go through all of those starvation and cleansing and cabbage and grapefruit and egg diets we've all tried? We chubs have had the will power; we just haven't had the correct guidance and information on how to take off the weight and keep it off and stay healthy all at the same time.

To show how pervasive the misinformation is, when I saw my gynecologist the other day and he complimented me on my weight loss, I proceeded to tell him how I did it. He said (as did a cardiologist friend of ours), "But pasta is good for you. Why, look at Greg LeMond, who cycled the Tour de France. He'd eat pasta before each race." So, I suggested to both of my colleagues that they give up medicine and start cycling all day so they could justify the pasta. Personally, I don't have the time or the inclination to cycle all day or exercise all day just so I can eat pasta.

Then he said to me, "I guess you are on mega vitamins?" I told him, "No, why should I be? I am eating healthier than I ever have. I need supplemental vitamins less than ever; I am getting them naturally by eating vitamin-rich food."

What is sad is that even health professionals have been convinced that pasta is good and nutritious and products like Special K cereal are good—because who can say that the cur-vaceously thin model in that commercial is anything but per-

U.S. WEIGHT GUIDELINES 1942–1995

QUICK, WHAT YEAR DO YOU WEIGH?

The first U.S. weight guidelines appeared in 1942 for women and in 1943 for men. Here are recommended weights since then for a woman 5 foot 6 and a man 5 foot 11.

	Woman 5'6"	Man 5'11"	Comments
1942–42	130–140	157–168	MET LIFE: all adults over 25: includes clothing and shoes
1959	124–139	147–163	MET LIFE: unclothed weights
1980	114–146	144–79	New federal guidelines
1983	130–144	152–165	MET LIFE: adults 25 to 59
1985	118–150	141–177	FEDERAL: women 19 to 25, subtract 1 pound each year under 25
1990	118–155 130–167	136–179 151–194	FEDERAL: both sexes, 19 to 34 Both sexes, 35 and up
1995	118–155	136–179	FEDERAL: both sexes

SOURCE: Copyright, January 8, 1996, U.S. News & World Report. Visit us at our Web site at www.usnews.com for additional information.

fect? Most cereals are loaded with sugar and they certainly are not healthy.

We have been given so much conflicting information that no one knows what is good, what is bad, which is saturated fat and which is nonsaturated fat, good fruit, bad fruit, no fruit, no alcohol, a little alcohol, pasta, multigrain bread and on and on. It really isn't that hard. All we have to do is decide if God made it or not. If God didn't make it, don't eat it. Plain and simple. Easy to measure. Easy to weigh. Easy to count. Easy to remember.

If we "cheat" once or twice a week (instead of five times a day), then that set point becomes easy to maintain. When you cheat, try eating only a bite or two of whatever it is that tempts you. You'd be surprised how well that works. Of course, not cheating at all is the healthiest way to live. However, let's get real. In this day and age, if we never had something "sinful" to eat, we'd lose out on a lot of fun in life. However, when we eat something sinful, we need to know that it is sinful. Once again, if God didn't make it, it must be sinful.

Now, does that mean that a piece of cake will never pass your lips again? No, it just means that you will start to make intelligent exceptions. If I eat something "bad" I know that the next day I will feel bloated and lethargic. If I really overdo it, I will have a "sick" headache during the night. I have learned to cheat a little, not cheat on multiple items. For example, if I

ARE YOU OVERWEIGHT?

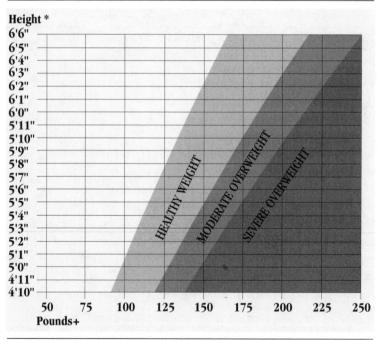

*Without shoes.

+Without clothes. The higher weights apply to people with more muscle and bone, such as many men.

SOURCE: Report of the Dietary Guidelines Advisory Committee on the "Dietary Guidelines for Americans," 1995, pages 23–24.

cheat on several items during the same meal, I'll feel miserable the next day. If I cheat during several meals on the same day, I will also feel miserable the next day.

I have learned to make the intelligent choice of whether feeling bloated and lethargic the next day is worth it. For example, my mother's homemade pie is worth it. Bread on my sandwich isn't. Even that pasta with Alfredo sauce isn't worth it. We are all different and we will all have different exceptions. **However, if you are trying to lose weight at this time, try not to make exceptions until after the weight is off.**

When I cheat, I gain 1 to 3 pounds overnight. Now, that is with only one item with one meal. Obviously, I am not cheating with 1 to 3 pounds' worth of calories. When I cheat, the sugar and flour cause me to bloat. That is why we can gain the weight so very fast. The sugar makes us retain water.

For example, if you are trying to lose weight, you will average 2 to 3 pounds per week with God's Diet. If you lose 2 pounds during the week, and then cheat with cake or wine on the weekend, you will gain back the weight overnight. You will get discouraged and think that the diet doesn't work. So, I highly recommend that no cheating is best until you have all the weight off.

I have also discovered that what some researchers have said about our "set point" is true. It is just that before I thought my set point was a lot higher. Now that I have lost my weight, I have found that my set point is 36 pounds less than I thought (or wanted to believe). After all, I wasn't chubby because I didn't have control, I was chubby because I had a higher "set point." Wrong, wrong, wrong. If we eat correctly, we will find our true set point. After I lost the weight, I was hoping that my set point was about 5 to 10 pounds less, but it isn't. I seem to maintain this weight no matter how much I eat from God's Diet. I don't lose more and I don't gain more (unless I cheat frequently).

Another wonderful side effect of eating correctly has been relief for people suffering from chronic headaches, people with migraines, people with PMS and allergies and fibromyalgia. When they follow the diet, the headaches are less frequent and in some cases go away altogether. I have seen the same thing with PMS. I have known for years, from personal experience, that when I got rid of the sugar in my diet, the PMS and cramps were better. Now I know why: when I got rid of the sugar I was not bloated. When I got rid of the sugar, I didn't crave the sugar.

For any of you who have PMS, you know you want sugars and chocolate more during that time than at any other time in the month. I maintain that if you get on God's Diet, then not only will your PMS be better, it may disappear. It is certainly worth a month or two of trying to see if you can get rid of the PMS and get control of your life during that difficult time (for your sake as well as for everyone around you!).

What about those of you who are already at your ideal weight? You get plenty of exercise and can eat anything you want. Your blood chemistry values are perfect, you feel great, and you know that your arteries are as clean as the day you were born. Go for it, eat everything. Don't bother to change. You have obviously mutated and evolved as the rest of us haven't. You are lucky and very much in the minority. There might even be days that I envy you, but not many. After all, it really isn't difficult to give up pasta and bread when you feel better without it and you know you are healthier without it.

It is very important to drink eight to ten 8-ounce glasses of water a day. Coffee and other caffeine drinks don't count. They act as diuretics and you can actually get mildly dehydrated if you drink too much caffeine. Water helps your body function. It helps to break down the stored fat and is also a by-product of fat catabolism (breakdown). You need water to keep every organ in your body working. Even if you eat 100 percent correctly, you will lose the weight very slowly if you don't have all the water you need.

Another important thing to remember is to eat three meals a day. When you go on a starvation diet, your body thinks it is in a time of deprivation. (Remember, you and I haven't evolved much from the days of the cave men—and they knew deprivation.) So, when we indicate to our bodies that we are in a time of starvation, our bodies start to fight to save us, thus preventing us from losing weight. If we make our bodies think that it is a time of plenty, by eating three meals a day, then we will actually lose more weight. Even if your life is hectic beyond comprehension, you can always grab some orange juice and a banana and have it on the way to work. For lunch, you can always order a burger and then throw away the bun and sweet pickles. Add a nice juicy apple for dessert. Cut it into pieces and eat it slowly for the most enjoyment. And remember, "An apple a day keeps the doctor away."

One of my theories on that saying ("An apple a day . . .") is that the apple is high in fiber and adds to better and more frequent bowel movements. Fuller and more frequent bowel movements are good. In fact, we should really be having a bowel movement after each meal, just as babies and puppies do. And while we are on this subject that most people find odious, let's really talk about it.

When we go to the doctor and are asked what our stool looks like or how frequently we go, most people get embarrassed and don't even know the answer. We know what we put into our bodies, but not much about the garbage we push out. As I tell my younger patients, you wouldn't want to live in your house if you didn't flush the toilet for a week. (I don't have any trouble tackling this subject with my older patients because they have realized how important a good bowel movement is. They've lived long enough to know how they feel if they don't have a bowel movement for a day or two.) Well, not having a bowel movement for several days is affecting your body the same way not flushing your toilet would affect your house. The stool acts as a poison and you get headaches and backaches, feel lousy, act lousy, and, worst of all, we know that if this becomes a chronic problem, you are more at risk for developing diverticulosis, diverticulitis, and colon and rectal cancer. Therefore, have an apple a day.

One of the jobs of the colon is to absorb the water from the food that is being processed on its way to the rectum. If you don't drink enough water, the colon will still do its job of pulling out the water from the sludge. If you don't drink enough water, then this sludge becomes too dry and hard. Hard rocks of stool do not send the same message to the brain as soft and full bowel movements. We don't get the urge to defecate as often when we have hard stools. So even if you eat all of the fiber in the world, you will still end up with constipation unless you drink enough water.

CHEATING

While cheating is realistic, as I've said before, you shouldn't cheat until after you've lost the weight. Otherwise, those bad foods will slow you down so much that you will get discouraged and give up.

We have all the great food that God made. When our diet is completely legal, we lose weight to our set point and stay at that set point. These foods are "perfect."

We also have foods such as cake. There is only one good thing about cake, and that's its taste! However, nutritionally it is lousy and we chubs gain weight eating it.

Then we have food like popcorn. Nutritionally, it is okay. However, we chubs will gain weight eating it. While I consider popcorn a cheat, it isn't as bad as a piece of cake. Hold off on popcorn and other foods on the swing list until after you've lost your weight.

As for corn flakes, not only has the outer coating been removed from the corn, and the shape drastically changed, but then lots and lots of sugar has been added. Don't even think about ever having corn flakes again.

Remember, counting calories doesn't work because 80 calories of celery is not equal to 80 calories of cake.

When you eat granulated fructose, you just absorb it—right now! No mess, no fuss, no good. Truly, a minute on the lips, forever on the hips. That's why I couldn't lose weight on an 800-calorie yogurt diet. All calories are *not* created equal.

꽃

To help you realize that caffeine is a drug and why I'd rather you not have any, please read the following side effects from caffeine: restlessness, excitement alternating with drowsiness, ringing in ears, fast pulse, nausea, increased urination, dehydration, thirst, tremor, delirium, convulsions, coma and then death in cardiovascular and respiratory collapse.[10] I hope none of us drinks so much as to cause all of these symptoms. However, the list of side effects should elicit new respect for this drug. We normally experience the increased urination with possible dehydration and the subsequent fatigue. So, by decreasing the caffeine you will be conserving the water, and you will have more energy.

Speaking of water, I have a suggestion for a quick and easy way to drink a few extra glasses of water every day. Each time you go to the bathroom, you also wash your hands. So, have one of those 4-ounce glasses handy and drink one of those afterward. You have just added another 16 ounces or more of water to your regime every day.

CHAPTER 3

VITAMINS, MINERALS, AND CHOLESTEROL

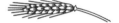

So, is this diet for everyone? No, but it is for almost everyone. We know there are lots of metabolic disorders that must have restrictions of certain foods and increased levels of other foods. When I have patients with diarrhea, I put them on clear liquids the first day—liquids high in simple sugars. Why? Because they need the sugars for easy and quick replacement of the calories and sugar they are losing so rapidly out of their system with the very act of having diarrhea. Early man didn't have Gatorade, Pedialyte, or IV fluids and so was more likely to die when he couldn't eat because of injury or illness.

If you are under medication or have a medical problem, you should check with your doctor to make sure that something God gave us won't be harmful to you.

Does this way of eating help diabetes and high cholesterol and triglycerides? It certainly appears to work. Later, I will show you case studies with lab work and weights before patients started to eat correctly and then again several months later. It becomes obvious that by just eliminating the simple carbos that God didn't make, cholesterol values go down, triglyceride values go down, the serum glucose values go down, as do weight and blood pressure. In fact, 93 percent of my God's Diet patients had their cholesterol and triglycerides go down. That's right 93 percent! I never got results like that from those so called "low-cholesterol diets." Now if I have a new patient with a lipid or glucose problem, I start him or her on God's Diet.

What about vitamins? If you eat a balanced diet—which is what God intended with the diversity of food he offered us— then you probably don't need any vitamins. All that money that you have been using for all of those supplements can be used to buy smaller clothes or put in the bank. Besides all of the other benefits of eating correctly, it is also cheaper. Packaged food is practically always more expensive than fresh food. If, however, you have a hard time eating a variety of foods and are stuck on just a couple of different fruits or vegetables, then take a multivitamin as a little insurance policy.

While a balanced diet should give us all of the vitamins and minerals we need, there is some concern that we are producing food from overused soil. Therefore, a vitamin and mineral supplement may help. However, anyone who thinks that having multiple vitamins, mineral supplements, and water is adequate nutrition is a pickle short of a full jar!

There is still so much we do not know about all of the herbal and alternative medicines. Those of us who practice Western medicine generally are not well schooled in alternative medicines or their usage, dosage, or side effects. We are just beginning to rediscover the many medicines that were known in the ancient days and learn how to use them. Do not be deceived, however. Whether it is a naturally grown herb being used as medicine or a laboratory concoction, it is still medicine, it is still a drug. "Natural" does not equal "good" and "harmless"—just look at cocaine and, for that matter, sugar!

With God's Diet, my patients' cholesterol and triglycerides

go down. If a patient's cholesterol still won't go down far enough, I would much rather have him try grapefruit fiber or fish oil for the triglycerides before we jump into the expensive and potentially liver-damaging medications that physicians are often forced to prescribe. Certainly those cholesterol and triglyceride values must come down! If we are smart we'll do whatever is necessary. However, I still feel that our whole lifestyle must change if we are to get back our national health.

We now have a non-fat fat. It is being used in potato chips, and it is hoped that by eating these chips instead of the standard chips, people won't be so fat. There is also a new drug on the market that will help keep fat from being absorbed from other foods in our diet. We will need to be much more cautious of vitamin deficiencies of the fat-soluble vitamins—A, D, E and K. I fear that we shall see people overeating the new potato chips and other non-fat food items and not only getting diarrhea, but subsequently developing vitamin deficiencies. The problem with these two "drugs" is that the fat we eat is not the enemy. Sugar is the enemy. When we start playing around with Mother Nature, we human beings are the ones most likely to get into trouble.

What about the starving people around the world—the ones dying of low caloric intake as well as of protein deprivation? Feed them the fortified high-caloric foods until they are well enough to start growing the foods that are healthy. After all, when you're ill or malnourished, you want to make things as easy on the body as you can. That is why Pedialyte and glucose-containing IVs came into being. The problem we have in more developed countries is that we *overeat* foods that are high in sugars. We eat all this sugar all the time. That is why we have so much high blood pressure, diabetes, high cholesterol, and high triglycerides.

I know, how can you eat fat and lower your cholesterol? I contend that it is the simple carbohydrates we eat, rather than the cholesterol we eat, that cause us to make the cholesterol.

We have all seen some of the more recent information that

says eggs aren't as bad as we've been told. I propose that what Dr. Robert Atkins said in *Dr. Atkins' Diet Revolution* in 1972 was right on target:

> Studies have shown that you cannot absorb more cholesterol than is in two eggs each day. More importantly, there is a feedback control mechanism in your body so that the more cholesterol you eat, the less you manufacture. And three-fourths of your body's cholesterol comes from what you manufacture yourself, usually from dietary carbohydrates.[11]

He also stated, ". . . in actual practice, cutting out carbohydrates on the diet lowers the cholesterol sometimes as much as 200 points." My statistics don't usually reveal such a high loss. However, my statistics show that 93 percent of my patients decrease their total cholesterol, triglycerides, and LDL (the bad cholesterol).

In fact, it was Dr. Atkins who was the initial inspiration for my diet. His diet worked, but it was just too hard to figure out how many carbos we could eat from which foods. We still had to weigh food and figure out the grams per ounce from a chart. With God's Diet, you don't need a single book, chart, or scale. If God didn't make it, don't eat it. It is really so simple, that when I originally used this with my patients, I didn't even write it down. I really couldn't understand that people needed more information than I was giving them orally. Not until one of my patients spent money at the bookstore getting a calorie counter and a book of "good" foods and a daily log, did I realize that I had to write something for my patients. I am probably on the eighth edition of that five-page handout, and that is what inspired me to write what you are presently reading. I can't keep this exciting and intelligent way of eating out of the hands of others by limiting it to the patients in my practice and the friends with whom they share it.

CHAPTER 4

CASE STUDIES

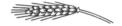

What good is a diet book without a few case studies? All of my patients have variations of the same story: "I've been on every diet in the world." "I always gain the weight back." "I am tired of being fat." "I am tired of people talking about me." "I really don't eat much." "I will sometimes just get overwhelmed with deprivation and eat every donut in sight." "I'm eating a 'balanced diet' and yet I can't lose the weight."

I think that one of our many mistakes is going on a "diet." When we use that term we are always thinking deprivation. It is time that we start thinking of the other definition of diet, which is a "habitual" course of living or, especially, feeding; hence, "food and drink regularly provided or consumed."[12] This is how I want you to interpret "God's Diet": as your habitual way of eating, not as a temporary state of doing without.

Some of these cases will refer to the use of Fastin and Pondimin. These pills were a godsend for many. I started prescribing them, reluctantly. I was *never* going to be a Diet Doctor. (Just goes to show you about never saying never.) However, I had so many people begging me for help, that I started using them. I discovered that they were not a panacea. The patient still had to be following a weight loss program, and he or she had to follow God's Diet if they were going to get the pills from me.

When the phen/fen (Fastin/Pondimin) drugs were pulled off the market, many patients just gave up. They felt they didn't have the willpower to change their eating habits without the pills. It was a tragedy for many. While possible serious side effects were always known, and even when it looked like there may be even more serious side effects for a few, the negative possibilities didn't even approach the known and almost universal side effects from obesity, such as hypertension and diabetes.

There isn't a single medicine (or herb or "natural medicine") that won't cause some side effect in some person. Our society must decide if the possible side effect is worth the risk.

For example, is Viagra worth a possible heart attack? To help prevent heart attacks and osteoporosis, is it worthwhile to take hormones even though there is a slightly increased risk of uterine and breast cancer? The rare side effect from taking polio vaccine or other vaccine and contracting the disease? Life is a risk. I'd rather give phen/fen to my patients who need it so they can eat properly rather than treat their high cholesterol with medication and then have to check their cholesterol every six weeks to make sure that I am not destroying their liver. I'd rather give someone a pill for the rest of his or her life to avoid diabetes than treat the diabetes after the fact.

If life were fair, none of us would be writing or reading this book, because we could all eat and drink and do anything we wanted and never suffer or cause any harm. But, God just didn't set it up that way, so we need to do the best we can to live and eat the way He set it up. If we need pills to eat correctly, or to treat a disease even if it is self-inflicted, then I guess it is all right to take those pills, since God gave us doctors and scientists to develop those pills.

So, now I'll get off my soapbox and get into those case studies.

CASE 1

It is only fitting that we start with the first patient who was actually on my program. The few patients who had participated before her had been given pills and had been told how to eat God's Diet in a less regimented way. It only took about three or four patients, all failures, before I realized that a specific program had to be used if I were going to really help anyone. So, this woman was the one.

She had been very active in Weight Watchers™ and had even been a lecturer. She followed "good nutrition" and yet didn't seem to be getting anywhere. She had become desperate to lose weight. She was becoming depressed about it. She was suffering terribly from her migraine headaches. (In fact, that is why she came to me in the first place. I am not sure why she came to me in the second place, because the injection I gave her for her migraine headache really made her sick.) At that time I had no idea that the new way of eating I was going to teach her would also solve her headache problem.

She wanted to lose 30 pounds and ended up losing 34 pounds. She usually walks her half hour every day. Her migraines disappeared. She feels great and eats great. Her triglycerides went from 96 milligrams/deciliters (mg/dl) to 67 mg/dl (Normal: 10–160 mg/dl) and her cholesterol from 211 mg/dl to 177 mg/dl (Normal: 120–200 mg/dl).

CASE 2

This next patient was shopping and overheard someone talking about the diet. My name was also mentioned. She called her mom and had her look up my name in the phone book.

(Luckily the person called me Dr. Gault instead of Dr. Dorothy, as most of my patients call me.) She came right over to the office that day and we started her new life that same day.

She was the patient who made me realize that I needed to write out the diet. We had all become so indoctrinated in counting and weighing everything, that to just change the way we eat to "God's Diet" was actually a hard concept for many. So, she became the recipient of the first edition of the God's Diet handout.

She had slowly gained weight over the years. She wasn't really upset with her weight and didn't really plan on losing it—until that day in the store when she heard my name. Since then, she has come weekly to weigh in and get a little verbal boost. She has been the most strict on the diet. Even when she found out she could have more than what she was eating, she did not indulge. If anything is packaged and has any chemical or preservative, she will not eat it. She is more of a purist than she has to be, but she's better off for going totally "God-given."

She also has a thyroid problem. Her endocrinologist was continually raising her Synthroid. She weighed 270 pounds when she came to me. She lost 64 pounds in 5 months. She has another 60 pounds to go. She dropped her Synthroid from 0.175 to 0.1 mg. Her cholesterol went from 169 to 164. She started walking a half hour every day and then became some-what overenthusiastic and began exercising three and a half hours a day. I don't encourage that much exercise, but it seems to make her happy. Who am I to say that exercising so much is bad for you? A hundred years ago all of us would have been in the fields working longer than three and a half hours a day. We need to keep reminding ourselves that this modern way of living really isn't all that it's cracked up to be. We have been sitting and eating our way into the grave.

She had been on phen/fen, though she never told her husband (as so many of my ladies didn't). She probably needed to be on pills for life because when phen/fen was pulled off the market, she went back to her old eating habits.

Before that, she had gone down from a size twenty-six dress to a size sixteen.

CASE 3

How could I write this without including my rather eccentric patient who went on the diet to lower her cholesterol and triglycerides just to prove me crazy? She just didn't believe that this way of eating was better for her triglycerides than a low-fat diet. She had been on lipid-lowering drugs, but we had to stop them because of the damage they were doing to her liver.

Once she started the diet, her triglycerides went from 503 to 223 and her cholesterol stayed stable (up 4 points) in only one month. However, she was displeased with the diet and went back to her "low-fat" muffins. Within another month her triglycerides went back up to 396 and her cholesterol only went down a few points. Subsequently, she returned to God's Diet.

CASE 4

This patient started at 190 pounds. She wants to weigh 125 pounds. She has lost 42 pounds in 6 months. Her cholesterol has gone from 223 to 171 and her triglycerides from 163 to 91. She lost her weight, sometimes with phen/fen and sometimes without, but always on God's Diet.

CASE 5

One woman lost weight faster than anyone. There is no particular reason. I know she rarely cheated, but then most of the successful patients have rarely cheated. She went from 218 pounds to 159 pounds (59 pounds) in 4 months. Her cholesterol decreased 50 points, from 184 to 134, and her triglycerides fell from 64 to 57. She walked about a half hour every day.

After losing a total of 91 pounds she was "graduated."

CASE 6

This sweet seventy-six-year-old woman had a weight problem for many years. She finally decided to do something about it because she had hypertension and diabetes. She put herself on a fat-free diet and lost about 17 pounds. I never talked to her about God's Diet. (I was still in the non-pushy stage.)

Subsequently, she came for one of her routine visits and was complaining about how itchy her skin was. She was literally scratching her skin raw. (Down here in the desert Southwest, we have a very dry climate and we have lots of dry skin and bloody noses from the dryness.) We tried several creams and several visits before I realized that her problem was possibly a lack of fat in her diet. I immediately switched her over to God's Diet. Her skin stopped itching and, as an extra bonus, she is no longer on medicine for her diabetes and we have decreased her blood-pressure medicines. She lost an additional 17 pounds and feels great.

CASE 7

This forty-two-year-old man decided he had to drop some of his 318 pounds, just weeks before his younger brother died of a massive heart attack. While his cholesterol and triglycerides were already in the normal range, he lost another 43 milligrams on his cholesterol and 12 milligrams on his triglycerides. He is more determined than ever to get the rest of the weight off and keep it off so that he won't meet his brother on the other side of the veil too soon. He's now down 50 pounds in three months.

CASE 8

This forty-six-year-old woman didn't want to start the diet until her life calmed down. She also didn't want to give up her bread. That was probably the hardest part for her. She finally went on God's Diet when lots of people at work were losing the weight and she wasn't. She lost 40 pounds in six months and her cholesterol decreased by 43 milligrams. Her triglycerides have gone down 61 milligrams. She feels great! She has only another 14 pounds to go.

CASE 9

This gal had been dieting and working out with a trainer. She was doing everything that he told her to do, but she wasn't losing weight and she was very discouraged. She thought she would never be able to weigh less. When she started eating God's Diet, she lost 11 pounds in four weeks. Her trainer can't believe it and neither can this patient. She is so encouraged that she really can weigh a more reasonable weight.

CASE 10 AND CASE 11

These are a mom and daughter. The mom came in at 298 pounds and has lost 31 pounds in ten weeks. The daughter started at 174 pounds and has lost 20 pounds in ten weeks. The daughter is losing more slowly than the mom, but that is probably because she doesn't have as much weight to lose. They are a delightful twosome and the husband/dad is delighted that his girls are finally eating healthily.

Since I first wrote about these two, the daughter hasn't lost much more weight, but she also hasn't gained it back. Mom, however, has continued to lose weight and as of this printing she has lost 125 pounds. She only has 21 more pounds to go.

CASE 12

This is a gentleman who came to me with a blood pressure of 168/114 and weighed 344 pounds and was only five feet six inches tall. In six months his weight is down 58½ pounds and his blood pressure is normal. The blood pressure medications I gave him on that first visit have long since been discontinued.

It seems that just eating correctly lowers the blood pressure faster than losing weight some other way.

CASE 13

This forty-five-year-old female went to see her physician and discovered she weighed 160 pounds at five feet five inches. She got scared that she was getting fat and decided to lose weight. She went on God's Diet and lost 33 pounds in three months.

CASE 14

This is probably my happiest story. I was doing a book signing and this lady came up to me just to thank me. Her son had elevated lipids since first being tested at the age of five. His cholesterol has been as high as 510 (normal is 120–200) and his triglycerides as high as 750 (normal is 10–150). The son is now fourteen years old. Eight months ago, his doctor was going to put him on lipid-lowering drugs. His mother decided to first try God's Diet. His cholesterol is now 153 and his triglycerides are down to 52. His HDL (the good cholesterol) was down to 30 and now is up to 64 (normal is greater than 35) and now he doesn't have to go on lipid-lowering drugs! Isn't that a great story?

CASE 15

One of the most exciting things a doctor can do is give someone back his or her health. Who would have ever thought that just being logical could make such a difference to so many people?

One of my patients weighed 218 pounds. She had been on a total of 50 units of insulin when she came to see me. She has only lost 13 pounds in three months, but she has been able to decrease her insulin to 8 to 10 units a day. What an exciting time in her life: to be taking less medicine, losing weight, and having more energy than she'd had in a long time.

CASE 16

This woman has fibromyalgia and lupus. Fibromyalgia and lupus are inflammatory illnesses of unknown cause. Fibromyalgia is characterized by pain, tenderness, and stiffness of muscles, tendon insertions, and adjacent soft-tissue structures. Lupus patients often complain of intermittent arthralgias, fever, and fatigue.[13] She also had a weight problem when she started God's Diet. She lost 28 pounds, which is wonderful all by itself. But what is even better is that if she doesn't cheat, her fibromyalgia and lupus seem to be in remission.

It really makes sense when you think about it. We are just killing ourselves with the way we are eating. When we eat all of this processed and sugar-loaded food, we can't help but mess up our bodies.

CASE 17

This thirty-six-year-old man came to me when he moved into town. He weighed 374 pounds at six feet tall. We discovered he had high blood pressure, diabetes, and hypothyroidism. We were treating all of those and he wouldn't even try to lose weight. Then he developed venous insufficiency and cellulitis in his legs. That got his attention and he finally decided to deal with the cause of so many of his problems.

He lost 77 pounds in thirteen months and we were able to take him off his medication for diabetes and lower his medication for hypertension. His legs cleared up and he is a much happier man.

CASE 18

This had been a colleague of mine who was always losing and gaining weight. I was helping his wife deal with depression and bulimia and, of course, had put her on God's Diet plus medication for depression. While she improved, so did her husband. When he came to the office with his wife one day, he told me he had lost 98 pounds and was down to his ideal weight, just by eating God's Diet.

CASE 19

I had a patient, a seventy-year-old gentleman, who was a *purist*. He never cheated and didn't eat anything that wasn't fresh or frozen. He lost 25 pounds in six months and his cholesterol went from 232 down to 109.

CASE 20

This thirty-two-year-old female e-mailed me that she loved the diet. She had gained 4 pounds, yet she felt healthier than she ever had. She wondered, though, why she gained weight instead of losing it. It took me several days to realize that she had been underweight and that by eating God's Diet her weight had gone back up to where it belonged.

This is a healthy way to eat. This is not a way to eat if you are interested in being pencil thin. God's Diet will get you to your true "set point."

❦

The moral to all of these cases and all of the other cases that I haven't included in these pages is: When you follow God's Diet,

1. you will achieve your true "set point."
2. lipids will decrease in 93 percent of the people.
3. allergies will get better.
4. migraines will get better or disappear.
5. blood pressure will normalize.
6. blood sugars will normalize—that includes both people with diabetes, who will need less medication, and people with hypoglycemia, who will stop having attacks.

7. you will have more energy than you've ever had.
8. fibromyalgia will improve.
9. your mood will improve.
10. your energy level will increase.
11. chronic headaches will improve.
12. heartburn improves.

I am sure that one day this list will be even longer as more and more people learn about this logical and intelligent way of eating.

CHAPTER 5

MENUS

This way of eating is for the *entire* family—even children on baby food. You wouldn't give children alcohol—it's poison, nor coffee—so why would you give them all that sugar? We give them sandwiches because it's easy—but it sure isn't healthy. For baby food for the little ones, just put the carrots or other food in a blender. You'll have natural, freshly cooked food without all those preservatives.

So, what about some sample menus? Not a problem. These are just examples. Please do not follow these as if they were gospel and the only things to eat on certain days. If you do that, then you haven't paid attention. Please, be creative. Don't limit yourself. Eat three meals a day. If you skip meals, your body thinks it is starving and your metabolism will actually slow down. If you don't have time for a meal, at least grab a piece of fruit or a veggie and eat it raw and on the run. Don't let your body think it is being deprived or it will try to sabotage your weight loss.

⊸ BREAKFAST ⊶

a bowl of fresh fruit

OR

a small glass of orange juice (preferably freshly squeezed. Tropicana and Minute Maid both have a freshly squeezed version.)

a bowl of Nabisco Shredded Wheat–usually with fruit such as a banana, strawberries, or raspberries on top–with milk

OR

two or three scrambled eggs made with mushrooms and cheddar cheese and a little salsa on top to spice it up

bacon

glass of tomato juice

add a parsley sprig for color

The last menu is obviously made when you have a day off and feel like spending a little more time in the kitchen.

⊸ LUNCH ⊶

Because my day is so hectic and we don't have a set time nor length of time to eat, I usually have two to three pieces of fruit and/or vegetables, depending on the time of year and what is available. During the winter I am especially fond of apples; I slice them into wedges and eat them between patients' visits. I love melons and plums and grapes and nectarines. I love to buy those little packages of peeled baby carrots—a perfect food to eat on the run. I really like buying cucumbers and peeling them and eating them like a banana. If I am in the mood for a salad, I buy the prepackaged bags of salad and just add my salad dressing. (As you can see, I don't spend a lot of time cooking and worrying about exotic meals. If you have the time, go for it. If you don't, there is no need to be deprived; just buy the food already cleaned and cut.)

OR

Salads

OR

Gazpacho

OR

Soup

OR

Leftovers from last night's dinner

DINNER

Salad of apple chunks with pieces of chopped nuts and dates on a bed of spinach leaves

Steak

Baked potato with butter and sour cream

Green beans

Fruit and cheese for dessert (if you need dessert to feel complete)

OR

Salad of shredded lettuce with banana and fresh pineapple slices

Pork chops with sugar-free apple sauce

Broccoli with cheese sauce

Brown rice

OR

Ham

Baked sweet potatoes

Brussels sprouts

Tossed salad with Marie's Blue Cheese Dressing

OR

Salad of Diet Jell-O with raspberries

Baked chicken (yes, you can even eat the skin)

Mashed potatoes

Steamed carrots

For the average dinner, I suggest a piece of meat, fish, or fowl with two veggies.

CHAPTER 6

RECIPES

Now for a bunch of recipes. I pulled these from my own recipe box as well as from friends, from family, and from recipe books. If other than from my own recipe box (which came mostly from my mother, Alice Gault, my grandmother, Jennie Pedersen, and my sister, Florence Schetgen), I'll give credit where credit is due. Once again, be creative. Just because I might like something and include it, doesn't mean you'll like it. You know the mantra: If God didn't make it, don't eat it. Therefore, if God didn't make it, don't bother cooking with it, either.

When you read the recipes that follow, don't expect them to specify BROWN rice or LEGAL (that is, no sugar, flour, corn syrup, or cornstarch has been added) sour cream. You need to realize that white is never the color of our rice and that there is no kind of sour cream you're going to use *except* LEGAL. When the recipe calls for anything that is canned, bottled, or packaged in any way, I mean the LEGAL equivalent. I may, however, add LEGAL to an ingredient if I think you may not be aware that it is often contaminated. Always read the labels. I was eating this way for a year before I realized that the manufacturers often add sugar to canned vegetables!

For those of you who keep a recipe box, we will be skipping right through Biscuits, Breads, Cakes, Candy, and Cookies.

➤ SALADS ➤

⟨⟩ CRAB SALAD

½ cup vinegar

4 packets Equal

2 stalks celery

1 green pepper

¼ bunch parsley

1 cup sliced, fresh mushrooms

1 pound crabmeat (or whitefish), picked over

First prepare the dressing by dissolving the Equal in the vinegar. Then cut up and marinate the vegetables in the dressing for approximately 30 minutes.

Toss the crabmeat lightly with your hands (freshly washed, of course). Pour a small amount of dressing over the crabmeat and mix. Use only as much dressing as needed. Add the marinated vegetables and refrigerate.

Before serving pour off any settled dressing.

MAKES 4–6 SERVINGS

∼ SIX-CUP SALAD

1 cup mandarin oranges (well rinsed)
1 cup pineapple tidbits (well rinsed)
1 cup coconut (LEGAL)
1 cup nuts (LEGAL)
1 cup whipping cream, whipped
1 cup sour cream

Combine all the ingredients and serve immediately or refrigerate for later use. Is best if used the same day it is made.

MAKES 4–6 SERVINGS

∼ JELL-O SALAD

1 16-ounce package diet lime Jell-O
1 9-ounce can crushed pineapple and juice (LEGAL)
1 cup whipping cream, whipped
1 cup mashed bananas
2 tablespoons freshly squeezed lemon juice

Prepare the Jell-O using hot water only. When dissolved, whip for 2 minutes. Add the pineapple and juice and the whipping cream.

Stir the lemon juice into the mashed bananas. Add to the Jell-O mixture and combine well.

Refrigerate until set.

MAKES 6–8 SERVINGS

❧ TOMATO ASPIC SALAD

5 cups tomato juice
3 3-ounce packages diet lemon Jell-O
2 teaspoons salt

Prepare the Jell-O with the tomato juice instead of water. Stir in the salt. Pour into a mold and chill.

MAKES 8–10 SERVINGS

❧ KIDNEY BEAN SALAD

1 16-ounce can kidney beans (rinse)
2 stalks celery, chopped
1 onion, chopped
vinegar to taste
water to taste
Equal to taste

Combine all the ingredients and refrigerate until the flavors are well blended.

MAKES 4–8 SERVINGS

❧ APPLESAUCE SALAD

1 6-ounce package lemon or lime diet Jell-O
1 tablespoon freshly squeezed lemon juice
1 cup homemade (or non-contaminated) applesauce

Prepare the Jell-O according to the package directions, decreasing the amount of water by 1 cup. Add the lemon juice and the applesauce. Mix well. Refrigerate until set.

MAKES 2–4 SERVINGS

⌘ TRANSYLVANIAN SALAD

(Harry Johnson, M.D.)

2 cucumbers
1 green pepper
1 bunch radishes
1 bunch green onions
1 cup mushrooms
4 tomatoes
oil
vinegar
mustard
salt and pepper

Dice the vegetables and place in a large bowl. Make a lot of sauce with the oil, vinegar, and mustard. Add salt and pepper to taste. Mix well and pour over the vegetables. Let stand at least overnight in the refrigerator to let the flavors meld.

This salad is to be made without lettuce, and all of the veggies should be fresh, not canned. Any veggie you want can be added.

MAKES 4–6 SERVINGS

ᔥ FRESH GREEN SALAD WITH ORANGE SEGMENTS AND FAT-FREE HONEY DRESSING

(Luanne Greenberg)

¼ *cup water*
¼ *cup red wine vinegar*
¼ *cup honey*
2 *heads of butter lettuce, leaves separated and washed*
1 *head of radicchio, leaves separated and washed*
2 *oranges, peeled and separated into segments*

Combine the water, vinegar, and honey in a small jar; cover and shake to mix ingredients. Arrange lettuce and radicchio on 6 salad plates. Divide orange segments among the salad plates; drizzle each with dressing.

MAKES 6 SERVINGS

ᔥ SAUERKRAUT SALAD

(Lois Tyler)

1 *quart sauerkraut (drained)*
1 *green bell pepper, diced*
1 *medium onion, diced*
1 *cup diced celery*
1 *small jar of pimentos, diced*
13 *teaspoons (39 packets) Equal*
½ *cup oil*
½ *cup vinegar*

In a large bowl, combine the sauerkraut with the vegetables.

In a medium bowl, whisk together the Equal, oil, and vinegar to make a dressing.

Pour the dressing over the sauerkraut mixture and let stand in the refrigerator overnight or even for a few days. Stir occasionally to blend the flavors. The salad will keep two weeks in the refrigerator.

MAKES 6–10 SERVINGS

⪼ WILTED LETTUCE WITH BACON DRESSING

6 slices bacon
⅓ cup vinegar
⅓ cup water
1 package Italian dressing mix
½ cup chopped green onions
4 teaspoons Equal
1 large head of lettuce, torn into bite-size pieces

Fry the bacon until crisp. Remove the bacon from the pan and drain off most of the grease. Add the vinegar and water to the pan. Bring to a boil. Add the Italian dressing mix and the green onions. Return to a boil. Remove the pan from the heat and then add the Equal.

Pour the dressing over the lettuce while hot. Crumble the bacon and sprinkle it on top.

> Don't heat Equal, because it may get a bitter taste. Always add artificial sweeteners after the heating is finished.

MAKES 6–10 SERVINGS

❧ JELL-O MOLD

3-ounce package diet lime Jell-O
1 small (4-ounce) package cream cheese, softened to room
  temperature and cut into cubes
1 small can crushed pineapple
1 small can Pet milk, whipped
½ cup chopped nuts

Prepare the Jell-O mix as instructed on the package and chill until almost set and still syrupy. Add the additional ingredients and whip until blended. Pour into Jell-O mold. Chill until set.

MAKES 6–10 SERVINGS

❧ STRAWBERRY JELL-O MOLD

1½ cups boiling water
1 3-ounce package diet lemon Jell-O
1 4-ounce package cream cheese, softened
1 cup whipping cream, whipped
1 3-ounce package diet strawberry Jell-O
1 cup boiling water
1 16-ounce package frozen strawberries, defrosted

Lightly oil a Jell-O mold or bowl. Chill the mold for 1 hour.

In a medium bowl, add the 1½ cups boiling water to the lemon Jell-O. Stir to dissolve the Jell-O. Chill just until the Jell-O becomes syrupy but not set. Using a hand mixer, whip the Jell-O.

Add the cream cheese and whipped cream to the Jell-O and blend well. Chill until set.

In a medium bowl, prepare the strawberry Jell-O with the cup of boiling water. Stir in the strawberries. Pour the mixture over the chilled lemon mixture and chill until set.

MAKES 6–10 SERVINGS

BLACK BEAN, CORN, AND BELL PEPPER SALAD

(Joyce Loudder)

½ pound black beans, soaked overnight

1 10-ounce package frozen corn, thawed

1 green bell pepper, chopped

1 red bell pepper, chopped

1 jalapeño pepper, seeded and chopped

3 green onions, sliced thin

2 tablespoons minced fresh cilantro

⅛ teaspoon salt

2 tablespoons olive oil

3 tablespoons freshly squeezed lime juice

Freshly ground black pepper to taste

Lettuce leaves (optional)

Drain the beans and cover with fresh water; cook for 1 hour or until tender. Cool the beans and drain.

Combine the beans, corn, green and red bell peppers, jalapeño pepper, green onions, cilantro, and salt. Add the olive oil and lime juice. Grind black pepper generously over the salad. Mix well. Serve on lettuce leaves, if desired.

This salad offers a brilliant palette of colors. Try serving it in hollowed-out tomatoes topped with a sprig of cilantro.

MAKES 6 SERVINGS

SOUPS

⤞ GAZPACHO

(Jack Bradley)

1 can stewed tomatoes, or fresh equivalent
1½ cups tomato juice without sugar
1 cucumber with or without peel, chopped
1 bunch of green onions, chopped
3 celery stalks, chopped
2 bell peppers, chopped
1 avocado, chopped
1 garlic clove, minced
¼ cup olive oil
2 tablespoons vinegar
1 teaspoon salt
½ teaspoon pepper
Tabasco sauce to taste
Freshly squeezed lime juice to taste

In a large bowl, mix all the ingredients and stir well. Refrigerate 24 hours before serving cold.

This is a cold soup that requires no cooking. It tastes better after the flavors have blended for 24 hours in the refrigerator. Try adding jicama and other veggies.

MAKES 4–6 SERVINGS

Jack eats this practically every day. Frankly, I thought he was a little nuts when he told me—until I made it. I must have had it practically every day for lunch for the next six months—obviously, not the original batch! The gazpacho stays fresh in the refrigerator for at least two to three weeks. So, if you don't know what to take to work for lunch, whip up a huge batch of this and you won't have to worry about lunch until you finally run out of it. I bought a food processor so that the cutting and chopping is now the easy and fun part. The hard part is the cleaning of the veggies.

✎ CHICKEN BROTH

1 4- to 5-pound chicken
12 cups cold water
5 celery stalks, with leaves
½ bay leaf
½ cup chopped onion
½ cup chopped carrots
6 parsley sprigs
1 teaspoon salt

In a large pot, cover the chicken with the water. Bring to a boil, then reduce the heat and simmer for 2 hours, skimming the top occasionally.

Add the remaining ingredients and simmer the chicken for 1 hour longer, or until it is tender. Add more salt if needed.

Let the chicken cool in the broth. Remove the chicken for another use. Remove the grease and chill the broth. It will thicken and make a good aspic.

MAKES ABOUT 6 CUPS

VEGETABLE SOUP

1 soup bone with meat
2 tablespoons shortening
4 cups hot water
½ bay leaf
3 peppercorns
1 medium onion, chopped
1 cup sliced carrots
1 cup sliced celery and leaves
1 (1-pound) can tomatoes
3 parsley sprigs, minced
1 tablespoon salt
¼ teaspoon crushed marjoram
¼ teaspoon thyme

Cut the meat off the soup bone and cut into small chunks. In a large pot, brown the meat in hot shortening. Add the water and the bone; cover and simmer 1½ to 2 hours.

Remove the bone and skim fat from the top of the soup. Place the ½ bay leaf and the peppercorns in a tea ball or tie in a cheesecloth bag; add to the soup. Add the remaining ingredients; cook 20 to 30 minutes longer, or until the vegetables are tender. Remove the tea ball or cheesecloth bag before serving.

MAKES 4 SERVINGS

❧ CHICKEN SOUP

(Laurie Jensen)

1 chicken, cut up
2 chicken bouillon cubes (I'm still looking for a LEGAL brand)
⅛ teaspoon salt
⅛ teaspoon pepper
¼ teaspoon dried basil
4 carrots, peeled and sliced
½ pound peeled boiling onions
2 teaspoons chopped flat-leaf parsley

Place the chicken pieces in a Crock-Pot. Cover with water. Add bouillon, salt, pepper, and basil. Simmer on low heat until the chicken is tender, about 1 to 1½ hours.

Remove the chicken from the stock and skim the excess fat. Bring the stock to a boil at 275°F. and add the carrots and onions. Lower the heat to 180°F. and simmer for 45 minutes.

Remove the skin and bones from the chicken, leaving the meat in large pieces. Return the chicken to the stock during the last 10 minutes. Sprinkle with parsley to serve.

MAKES 6–8 SERVINGS

☞ CALDILLO

(Alaine Bracken and Betty Burke)

1½ pounds cubed beef
½ teaspoon to 1 tablespoon chili powder
1 10-ounce can beef bouillon
1 10½-ounce can stewed tomatoes
2 cups boiling water
1 large onion, chopped
1 to 2 green chilies (depending on taste), chopped
1 garlic clove, minced
½ bunch of fresh cilantro or ½ teaspoon dried cilantro
3 medium tomatoes, cubed

In a large skillet, brown the cubed beef and add the chili powder. Cook for a few minutes longer.

Place the meat and the remaining ingredients into a Crock-Pot and cook for 8 to 10 hours. Start on high for 1 hour, then turn down to low for the remainder of the time.

MAKES 6–8 SERVINGS

☞ EASY SOUP

(Nancy Nance)

1 pound ground beef
1 16-ounce package frozen mixed vegetables
1 to 2 cups salsa

Mix all of the ingredients in a Crock-Pot. Cook for 4 to 5 hours on high and serve.

MAKES 4–6 SERVINGS

❧ SPLIT-PEA SOUP

1-pound package green split peas
6 or 7 cups cold water
1 ham bone (cooked or uncooked) or 1 smoked pork butt
2 carrots, sliced
2 medium onions, sliced
2 celery stalks, chopped
1 bay leaf
Salt and pepper

Wash and drain the split peas. Place them in a large pot, cover them with the water, and put in the ham bone. Bring to a boil, then reduce the heat and simmmer for 2 hours.

Add the vegetables and seasoning and bring to a boil again. Reduce the heat and simmer for 2 more hours, stirring frequently. (The soup will burn easily as the mixture begins to thicken.)

MAKES 6–8 SERVINGS

ENTRÉES

CHILI CON CARNE

> 1 to 2 tablespoons butter
> 4 to 5 onions, sliced
> 1 pound ground round steak
> 1½ teaspoons salt
> 1 tablespoon chili powder
> 1 12-ounce can tomato puree
> 1 cup water
> 1 2-pound can kidney beans (without sugar), well rinsed

In a large skillet, melt the butter. Add the onions and cook until tender but not brown. Remove the onions to a Dutch oven.

In the skillet, brown the meat, stirring and chopping to break up any lumps. When the meat is hot, add the salt and chili powder and simmer 20 to 30 minutes.

Add the meat mixture to the onions. Add the tomato puree and the water and bring to a boil. Add the beans, heat through, and serve.

MAKES 4–6 SERVINGS

PHEASANT WITH SOUR CREAM

> 1 pheasant, quartered
> 1 tablespoon butter
> ½ pint of sour cream
> 1 onion—chopped

Brown the pheasant in a skillet with butter at medium heat. Place the browned bird in a roasting pan. Mix the sour cream and onion with the fat in the skillet and then pour over the bird. Cover the roasting pan.

Place in a 350°F. oven for 45 minutes. Use the sour cream mixture as the gravy.

MAKES 4 SERVINGS

❧ CHICKEN CASSEROLE

> ½ cup chicken broth or milk
>
> 1 cup sour cream
>
> 3 cups diced cooked chicken
>
> 1 cup diced celery
>
> 1 can (8 ounces) mushrooms, drained
>
> 1 jar (2 ounces) pimentos, drained
>
> 1 can (8 ounces) sliced water chestnuts, drained
>
> ⅓ cup toasted almonds, sliced

Preheat the oven to 325°F.

In a large bowl, mix the broth with the sour cream, chicken and celery. Add the remaining ingredients and mix well. Lightly grease a casserole dish with vegetable oil. Pour the mixture into the casserole dish, sprinkle with the toasted almonds, and bake for 40 minutes.

MAKES 8–10 SERVINGS

⇜ LENTIL BURGERS

> 2 cups lentils
> 4 cups water
> 1 medium onion, chopped fine
> Salt to taste
> ½ teaspoon ground sage, or to taste
> Water
> Olive oil or cooking spray
> 1 to 2 cups rolled oats

Bring the water to a boil and add the lentils. Reduce the heat to a simmer and cover. Cook for 40 minutes or until tender. Drain.

In a medium bowl, combine the lentils, onion, salt, sage, and water. The mixture will be pasty.

Lightly coat a frying pan with oil. Add the lentil mixture and cook until the lentils are tender. Let the mixture cool, then form it into patties. Roll each patty in oats and fry in olive oil until heated through.

MAKES 4–6 BURGERS

⇜ ORIENTAL SHRIMP

> ¼ cup vegetable oil
> 32-ounce package frozen cleaned shrimp, defrosted, rinsed, and patted dry
> 1 onion, sliced thin
> 1 cup pineapple chunks
> ½ cup vinegar
> 2 tablespoons soy sauce
> 1 teaspoon dry mustard
> Equal to taste

In a large skillet, heat the oil. Add the shrimp and stir-fry for 5 to 7 minutes, until shrimp are opaque. Remove the shrimp from the pan and keep them warm.

To the skillet add the onion, pineapple, and vinegar. Bring to a boil. Season with the soy sauce and dry mustard. Cook 1 minute. Return the shrimp to the pan briefly to heat through in the sauce. Remove the pan from the heat and stir in the Equal. Serve over rice.

MAKES 6–8 SERVINGS

⋘ CHICKEN CASHEW CASSEROLE

1 cup mushrooms, sliced

½ cup water, chicken broth, or milk

2 cups sour cream

1 cup diced celery

¼ cup chopped onion

1 can of sliced water chestnuts, drained

3 cups diced cooked chicken (or tuna)

1 jar (2 ounces) pimentos, drained and chopped

¼ pound cashews, split

Preheat the oven to 350°F.

In a large bowl, combine all the ingredients. Turn into a lightly greased casserole and bake for 40 minutes, or until the vegetables are tender and the sauce is hot.

MAKES 4–6 SERVINGS

✥ BEEF STROGANOFF

(Madeline Anderson)

1 pound beef tenderloin cut 1 inch thick
1 garlic clove, cut in half, or a pinch of garlic powder
1½ teaspoons salt
¼ teaspoon pepper
4 tablespoons (½ stick) butter
½ cup minced onion
½ cup water
1 pound mushrooms, sliced
1 can cream of chicken soup (undiluted)
1 cup sour cream
Cooked rice
Chopped parsley, chives, or dill for garnish

The day before serving, trim fat off the meat. Rub garlic on both sides of the meat. Combine the salt and pepper and pound into both sides of the meat. Cut the meat into 1½- to 2-inch strips.

In a large skillet, heat the butter. Add the beef in batches and brown, turning often. Remove the meat and refrigerate.

In the same butter, sauté the onion until golden brown. Add the water and stir to dissolve any brown bits. Add the mushrooms and the soup and cook uncovered over low heat about 20 minutes, stirring occasionally, until the mixture is thickened. Remove from the pan and refrigerate.

The next day, about 20 minutes before serving, combine the beef with the mushroom mixture and the sour cream. Cook over low heat about 20 minutes or until heated through. Do not boil. Serve over rice. Sprinkle with parsley, chives or dill.

MAKES 6–8 SERVINGS

✒ BROILED LAMB SHISH KEBAB

(Royal Caribbean Cruise Line)

6 white onions
2 green bell peppers, cut into squares
2 red bell peppers, cut into squares
3½ pounds lean lamb, cut in cubes
2 cups olive oil
Lemon juice from 4 lemons
2 bay leaves
Salt and pepper to taste
1 bunch of parsley, chopped
Pine nuts, toasted for garnish (optional)

Slice 2 of the onions into squares similar in size to the peppers. Finely chop 3 of the onions and press to save the onion juice. Discard the onion solids. Reserve the remaining 1 onion.

Place the lamb cubes in a medium bowl. In a separate bowl, blend the olive oil, onion juice, lemon juice, and bay leaves together. Season with salt and pepper. Pour the marinade over the lamb, making sure to completely cover all of the lamb. Place in the refrigerator overnight.

To cook the shish kebab, alternately thread lamb, peppers, lamb, and onion on bamboo skewers until each skewer is full. Heat a sauté pan to medium heat. Place a few skewers in the pan and cook, turning each skewer to brown all four sides. When cooked, place each skewer on a bed of rice.

Slice the remaining raw onion and mix with the chopped parsley. Garnish the skewers with mixed sliced onion and parsley and toasted pine nuts.

MAKES 6 SERVINGS

❧ MEDALLIONS OF PORK TENDERLOIN

(Royal Caribbean Cruise Line)

3 pounds pork tenderloin
½ teaspoon salt
⅓ teaspoon white pepper
6 tablespoons (¾ stick) unsalted butter
2 ounces chopped shallots
1½ cups veal brown stock
½ cup heavy cream
8 ounces seedless grapes
½ ounce parsley, chopped

Cut the pork tenderloin into 3-ounce portions and season with salt and white pepper.

In a large skillet, melt 3 tablespoons of the butter. Add the pork and sauté until no longer pink, about 4 minutes per side. remove the pork from the pan and set aside, covered to keep warm.

In the same skillet, melt 2 tablespoons of the butter and sauté the shallots for 2 minutes. Deglaze the pan with the brown stock, bring to a boil, scrape the bottom of the pan to dissolve all the drippings from the pork, and reduce the stock by half.

Add the cream, reduce the sauce further, and adjust the seasoning. Return the pork to the sauce and heat through.

In a small skillet, melt the remaining tablespoon of butter. Add the grapes and sauté until softened. Place 2 of the pork medallions on each dinner plate; put 4 or 5 grapes on top, then pour sauce over and around the pork and garnish with the parsley.

MAKES 8 SERVINGS

◈ LAMB ESTOFADO CONQUISTADOR

(Royal Caribbean Cruise Line)

½ cup vegetable oil
4 pounds lamb shoulder, bone removed, diced
4 tablespoons (½ stick) unsalted butter
1 cup chopped garlic
4 ounces finely chopped onions
1 cup guava juice (see note)
1 cup clear stock or bouillon
1 teaspoon salt
2 ounces green chili peppers, chopped
1 cup tomato paste
1 ounce cilantro, chopped

In a large skillet, heat the oil and sauté the diced lamb until well browned on all sides. Discard the fat and set the lamb aside.

In the same skillet, add the butter and sauté the garlic and onions briefly. Add the guava juice, stock, and salt and bring to a boil. Add the lamb. Cover and let simmer for 40 minutes.

Add the chili peppers and tomato paste and stir well. Cover and simmer for an additional 10 to 15 minutes, adjust seasoning, and sprinkle with cilantro.

The original recipe calls for guava nectar, but that contains lots of added sugar. Try to get guava juice and then add some honey. If you can't find guava, it should still taste wonderful with pineapple or other juice. We just won't tell the Royal Caribbean chef!

MAKES 8 SERVINGS

❧ RED SNAPPER A LA VERA CRUZANA

(Royal Caribbean Cruise Line)

8 6-ounce red snapper fillets
½ cup freshly squeezed lemon juice
½ cup freshly squeezed lime juice
½ cup fish stock (fat free)
2 cups chopped onion
2 celery stalks, chopped
1 cup chopped green bell pepper
2 garlic cloves, chopped
⅔ cup tomato paste
4 cups diced fresh tomatoes with juice
1 tablespoon capers
1 to 2 small jalapeño peppers
2 teaspoons oregano
1 bunch of cilantro, chopped
8 slices of lime

In a glass dish, marinate the fish in the lemon and lime juices for about 30 minutes.

Meanwhile, in a large skillet bring the stock to a boil. Add the onion, celery, green pepper, and garlic. Simmer 15 to 20 minutes, until tender. Reduce the heat and add the tomato paste, tomatoes, capers, jalapeño peppers, and oregano. Cook until slightly reduced.

Place the fish in the pan with the sauce. Simmer 15 to 20 minutes, until the fish is opaque. Place a fillet on each plate and sprinkle with cilantro. Garnish with a slice of lime.

MAKES 8 SERVINGS

⇾ DICK'S FAVORITE CASSEROLE

1 2-pound canned precooked ham, cubed
1 8-ounce can sliced water chestnuts, drained
1 4-ounce jar pimentos, drained and chopped
1 8-ounce can mushrooms
6 to 12 hard-boiled eggs, peeled and sliced
LEGAL mayonnaise to taste
3 celery stalks, sliced

In a large bowl, combine all the ingredients. Cover and refrigerate until ready to serve. (The casserole tastes even better the next day, after the flavors meld.)

MAKES 6–8 SERVINGS

⇾ CHICKEN CASSEROLE

(Sally Beyers)

4 cups cooked chicken, cubed
1 8-ounce can of sliced water chestnuts, drained
½ cup slivered almonds
1 cup mayonnaise (LEGAL)
1 4-ounce can mushroom pieces
2 teaspoons diced onions
½ cup cheddar cheese, shredded

Preheat the oven to 450°F.

Mix all the ingredients except the cheese in a casserole dish. Sprinkle with the cheese and bake for 30 minutes, or until the cheese is melted.

The casserole can be served as a hot or cold dish.

MAKES 4–6 SERVINGS

❧ FESTIVE CHICKEN

(Karen and Mike Crow)

2 tablespoons vegetable oil
1 medium onion, chopped
1 small green bell pepper, cut in julienne strips
1 garlic clove, minced
2 teaspoons curry powder
½ teaspoon dried thyme, crushed
¼ teaspoon ground cloves
1 16-ounce can tomatoes, cut up but not drained
¼ cup dried currants
½ teaspoon salt
1 2-pound broiler/fryer chicken, cut up
¼ cup sliced almonds, toasted
Hot cooked brown rice

In a deep frying pan or wok, heat the oil. Stir-fry the onion, green pepper, and garlic for 3 to 5 minutes, or until the onion is tender. Add the curry powder, thyme, and cloves and stir-fry 2 minutes longer. Stir in the tomatoes, currants, and salt. Add the chicken pieces, spooning tomato mixture over chicken. Bring to a boil, then reduce the heat. Cover and simmer for 35 to 40 minutes, or until the chicken is tender.

Remove the chicken; boil the sauce, uncovered, about 10 minutes, or until it is reduced to the desired consistency. Skim off any fat. Return the chicken to the pan and heat through. Garnish with toasted almonds and serve over rice.

MAKES 4–6 SERVINGS

❧ STEAK JAMAICAN

(Luanne Greenberg)

6 tablespoons honey
⅓ cup freshly squeezed lime juice
2 tablespoons vegetable oil
2 tablespoons prepared mustard
2 garlic cloves, minced
1 teaspoon grated lime zest
½ tablespoon salt
½ teaspoon coarsely ground black pepper
2 pounds lean top round steak
Lime wedges

In a small bowl, whisk together all ingredients except the steak and lime wedges. Score the steak across the top and place in a shallow baking pan. Pour the marinade over the steak; turn to coat all sides. Refrigerate 6 to 8 hours, turning occasionally.

Remove the steak from the refrigerator 30 minutes before cooking. Preheat the broiler. Broil the steak 4 to 6 inches from the heat source for 3 minutes per side for medium rare, or continue to cook to desired doneness. Slice thin on the diagonal. Serve with lime wedges.

MAKES 4–8 SERVINGS

✑ BEEF BRISKET

(Alaine Bracken)

4 whole green chilies (canned or roasted and freshly peeled),
*   diced*
Beef brisket
2 cans beef broth
2 to 3 cups boiling water

Place the green chilies in the bottom of a Crock-Pot. Cut the brisket to fit the pot. Add the beef bouillon and cover brisket with water. Cook on high for 6 to 8 hours.

MAKES 6–8 SERVINGS

✑ CASHEW CHICKEN

(Luanne Greenberg)

4 boneless, skinless chicken breasts, cubed
1 medium onion, diced
3 chicken bouillon cubes, crushed, or 3 teaspoons bouil-
*   lon granules*
3 cups (8 ounces) sliced mushrooms (or a 10-ounce can)
1 cup uncooked regular long-grain rice
2 teaspoons ground ginger
1½ cups boiling water (use less if chicken yields water
*   when cooking)*
2 cups broccoli pieces
1 cup cashew nuts
Salt and pepper to taste
Soy sauce to taste
Carrot shavings, for garnish

Preheat the oven to 375°F. In a 2½-quart round casserole dish, combine the chicken, onion, and one bouillon cube. Cover and microwave on medium high (70 percent power) for five minutes, stirring once. Add the mushrooms, rice, ginger, boiling water, and remaining bouillon cubes to the same dish. Cover and bake in the oven for 30 minutes.

Stir the casserole and add the broccoli, making sure the rice is covered with liquid. Bake another 10 minutes. If the vegetables are done to your liking, remove the casserole from the oven and let stand for a few minutes, so moisture will be absorbed.

Preheat the broiler.

Stir ½ cup of the cashews and the salt, pepper, and soy sauce into the casserole. Place the remaining cashews on top and put under the broiler (without the cover) to brown the top. Garnish with carrot shavings.

MAKES 4 SERVINGS

❧ CROCK-POT MEATLOAF

Make your favorite meatloaf recipe. Shape the meatloaf mixture into a round loaf and then center it in the Crock-Pot. Place halved potatoes and carrots around the meatloaf. Make a "gravy" with one can of cream of mushroom soup and one can of milk and pour over the meatloaf and vegetables.

Cook in the Crock-Pot on high for 6 to 8 hours.

MAKES 4–8 SERVINGS

❧ MEATLOAF

1 to 2 pounds ground beef
1 to 2 eggs
1 to 2 handfuls of rolled oats
Salt and pepper to taste

In a large bowl, combine all the ingredients, using clean hands.
Bake at 350°F. for 1½ hours or until done.

MAKES 4–8 SERVINGS

❧ PORK CHOPS

4 center-cut or loin pork chops
Salt and pepper
Vegetable oil
1 large onion, sliced into 4 thick slices
Applesauce

Season the pork chops with salt and pepper. Heat the oil in a
large skillet or electric frying pan and add the chops. Brown
the chops evenly, then top each with a slice of onion. Add
some water and tightly cover. Simmer for 45 minutes.

Serve with applesauce.

MAKES 4 SERVINGS

☞ SUNDAY POT ROAST

(Shellie Payne)

On Sunday morning (or any other morning, for that matter), season a roast and place it in the Crock-Pot. Peel and cut carrots and potatoes and place them on top of the roast. Add a little water. Cook on medium for 6 to 7 hours.

MAKES 6–8 SERVINGS

☞ RAINBOW TROUT

2 fresh whole rainbow trout, cleaned and gutted

2 tablespoons freshly squeezed lime juice

2 tablespoons melted butter

Dash of chili powder or cumin powder

Salt and pepper

¼ cup prepared tomato salsa

Lime wedges

Place the trout, flesh side up, in a microwave baking dish. Combine the lime juice and butter; drizzle over the trout. Season with chili powder, salt, and pepper; cover with wax paper. Microwave on HIGH for 3 minutes. Rotate the dish; cook 3 to 4 minutes longer, or until fish flakes with a fork.

Remove from the oven; top the trout with salsa and garnish with lime wedges.

MAKES 2 SERVINGS

☙ BAKED SALMON

4 to 6 salmon steaks, cut into slices
8 tablespoons (1 stick) butter, melted
2 tablespoons olive oil
1 teaspoon grated lemon zest
2 tablespoons freshly squeezed lemon juice
½ cup snipped fresh flat-leaf parsley
½ teaspoon seasoned salt
¼ teaspoon pepper
1 lemon, sliced

Arrange the salmon steaks in a single layer in a shallow baking dish. Combine the remaining ingredients, except lemon slices, and pour over the fish. Marinate for 30 minutes.

Preheat the oven to 350°F.

Baste the fish with the marinade, then top with the lemon slices. Bake for 20 to 25 minutes, or until the fish flakes easily with a fork.

MAKES 4–6 SERVINGS

⤳ CHICKEN DIVAN

(Pat Zamzow)

4 boneless chicken breasts with skin
Butter
2 10-ounce packages frozen broccoli spears
2 cans cream of chicken soup
½ to 1 cup mayonnaise
4 ounces shredded cheddar cheese
1 teaspoon freshly squeezed lemon juice
½ teaspoon curry powder
Hot cooked rice

Preheat the oven to 350°F.

Place the chicken breasts on a lightly buttered baking sheet. Cover loosely with a sheet of lightly buttered baking parchment or aluminum foil. Bake for 25 to 35 minutes, or until the chicken is done.

Meanwhile, prepare the broccoli according to the package directions. Drain.

In a small saucepan, heat the soup. Remove from the heat.

Remove the skin from the chicken and place the chicken in a 9 × 13-inch baking pan. Top with the broccoli.

Add the mayonnaise, cheese, lemon juice, and curry powder to the soup and blend well.

Pour the soup mixture over the chicken and broccoli. Bake 30 minutes, or until the sauce is bubbling. Serve with the rice.

MAKES 4 SERVINGS

❧ CHICKEN AND ASPARAGUS CASSEROLE

(Joy Guldeman)

> *2 tablespoons butter*
> *½ cup chopped onion (or more, to taste)*
> *¾ cup sliced celery*
> *1 pound trimmed asparagus, cut into 1-inch pieces*
> *4 cups cubed cooked chicken*
> *1 can cream of mushroom soup*
> *1 can cream of chicken soup*
> *½ can of water chestnuts, drained and chopped*
> *1 tablespoon freshly squeezed lemon or lime juice*
> *½ teaspoon curry powder*
> *1 cup mayonnaise*
> *½ cup shredded cheddar cheese*

Preheat the oven to 350°F.

In a medium skillet, melt 1 tablespoon of the butter. Add the onion and celery and cook until just tender, about 5 minutes. Set aside in a medium bowl.

In the same skillet, melt the remaining butter. Sauté the asparagus pieces until just tender, 5 to 7 minutes.

Arrange the chicken and the asparagus in the bottom of a 9 × 13-inch glass baking dish.

In the bowl with the onion and celery, combine the remaining ingredients except for the cheese. Pour over the chicken and asparagus. Sprinkle with cheese. Bake for 30 minutes, or until the cheese is melted and the sauce is bubbling.

MAKES 4 SERVINGS

◁≈▷ BARBECUED VEAL

3 slices bacon, diced
1 onion, diced
6-pound rolled leg of veal
Salt and pepper to taste
½ cup sour cream
1 small can of tomato puree

Preheat the oven to 300°F.

In a large skillet, cook the bacon and onion until the bacon is crisp and the onion is tender. Remove from the pan and set aside in a medium bowl.

In the skillet, brown the veal in the bacon fat. Place the veal in a roasting pan and season with salt and pepper.

Add the sour cream and tomato paste to the onion and bacon. Pour the sauce over the veal. Bake 3 hours, basting often.

MAKES 8–12 SERVINGS

◁≈▷ GLAZED CHICKEN

(Janet Bolser)

4 chicken breasts—boneless and skinless
Salt to taste
1 tablespoon of an all-fruit peach spread or all-fruit jam
⅓ cup sliced almonds, toasted

Salt the chicken and cook on medium heat in a nonstick skillet until the juices run clear, 10 to 12 minutes. Just before serving, add the peach spread to the warm pan, moving the chicken around until it is slightly coated. Garnish with almonds.

MAKES 4 SERVINGS

☙ POLYNESIAN CASSEROLE

(Madeline Anderson)

1½ pounds pork sausage
1 cup chopped onion
1 bunch of green onions with tops, sliced
1 green bell pepper, chopped
3 cups chopped celery
1 medium can mushrooms
3 flat-leaf parsley sprigs
1½ cups long-grain brown rice
2 cans chicken with rice soup
1 package slivered almonds

Preheat the oven to 300°F.

In a large skillet, brown the sausages. Remove them from the skillet, reserving the fat.

Add the onion, green onions, bell pepper, and celery to the skillet and cook until tender. Stir in the mushrooms and parsley and heat through. Stir in the rice, soup, and almonds.

Cut the sausages into 1-inch pieces and add to the vegetable mixture. Pour into a casserole dish, cover, and bake 2 hours.

MAKES 10 SERVINGS

⤷ STUFFED GRAPELEAVES

(Marsha Chanoux)

50 grape leaves (fresh or jarred)

BASIC STUFFING MIX
1 cup long-grain brown rice
1 pound lean ground beef or lamb, uncooked
1 to 2 tablespoons melted butter
Salt and pepper to taste
4 lamb bones
Salt to taste
3 lemons, peeled and juiced (peels reserved)

If you are using jarred leaves, rinse in cold water and squeeze thoroughly before rolling. If using fresh leaves, soak or steam them in boiling water about 15 minutes or until they are softened. Gently squeeze out the moisture and stem each leaf. Flatten each leaf and set aside.

Put the rice in a pan with 2 cups of water. Bring to a rolling boil and then drain. With your hands, mix the rice with the meat, butter, salt, and pepper to blend well.

Place about 1 tablespoon of stuffing in the center of each leaf. Fold the ends like an envelope and roll away from you cigar fashion.

Line the bottom of a large pot with the lamb bones. Arrange the leaves in rows, close together, alternating the direction of the rows with each layer. Sprinkle each layer with salt. Press down on the leaves with an inverted dish to tightly pack them. Add water to cover and bring to a boil. Reduce heat and simmer for 35 to 40 minutes. Add the lemon juice and peel. Simmer another 15 minutes before serving.

MAKES 10 SERVINGS

◆ PARTY MEATBALLS

(Judy Heater)

MEATBALLS

1½ pounds lean ground beef

½ cup rolled oats

1 tablespoon chopped flat-leaf parsley

½ teaspoon salt

⅛ teaspoon pepper

½ cup grated Parmesan cheese

2 eggs, beaten

2 tablespoons vegetable oil

SAUCE

1 garlic clove, minced

1 1-pound can tomatoes

1 6-ounce can tomato paste

1 teaspoon salt

⅛ teaspoon pepper

½ teaspoon oregano

¼ teaspoon basil

In a large bowl, combine all the meatball ingredients except the oil. Using a tablespoon, shape into small balls. In a large skillet, brown the meatballs in the oil, turning frequently to brown all sides.

Combine the sauce ingredients. Pour the sauce over the browned meatballs; simmer for 30 minutes. Turn into a chafing dish; keep hot.

MAKES 6–8 SERVINGS

VEGETABLES

QUICK BROCCOLI CASSEROLE
(Martha Poulos)

2 16-ounce packages frozen chopped broccoli
1 can cream of mushroom soup
¾ cup mayonnaise
2 eggs, well beaten
½ cup grated cheddar cheese
1 tablespoon butter, cut into small pieces

Preheat the oven to 350°F.

Cook the broccoli according to the package directions and drain well. Fold in the soup, mayonnaise, and eggs. Pour into a lightly buttered casserole and sprinkle with the grated cheese. Dot with the butter and bake for 30 minutes, until the cheese is melted and the sauce is bubbling.

MAKES 8–10 SERVINGS

PINTO BEANS
(Mittie Hudson)

4 cups pinto beans, washed and drained
Salt to taste (optional)
1 16-ounce jar picante sauce

Place the beans in a Crock-Pot and cover with water by at least 3 inches. Cook at least 8 to 10 hours. When the beans are tender and ready to eat, add the salt and picante sauce.

MAKES 8–12 SERVINGS

☞ MUSHROOMS

1 pound medium-size fresh mushrooms
2 tablespoons unsalted butter

Wash and trim the mushrooms and let them dry thoroughly. Place in the top of a double boiler with the butter. Steam for about 1 hour.

☞ CUCUMBERS

(Marlene Rowland)

2 large cucumbers, sliced thin
1½ teaspoons salt
1 cup sour cream
2 tablespoons freshly squeezed lemon juice
1 tablespoon finely chopped onion
2 tablespoons Equal
Dash of pepper
3 radishes, sliced
Lettuce leaves, washed and patted dry
1½ teaspoons finely chopped flat-leaf parsley

In a medium bowl, lightly toss the cucumbers with 1 teaspoon of the salt. Refrigerate until well chilled.

Combine ½ cup of the sour cream, the remaining ½ teaspoon of salt, and the remaining ingredients, except for the lettuce and parsley. Toss the cucumbers with the sour cream mixture and refrigerate.

Serve the salad on lettuce leaves with the remaining sour cream and the parsley, or serve it in a fancy dish and pass it around the table.

SIDE DISHES

⤳ CHILI CHEESE RICE

(Santa Teresa Country Club, Santa Teresa, New Mexico)

3 to 4 cups raw rice
2 cups sour cream
Salt to taste
½ pound Jack cheese, cut into 1-inch cubes
4 4-ounce cans chopped green chilies (or fresh green roasted chilies)
½ cup grated Jack cheese
1 tablespoon unsalted butter

Preheat the oven to 350°F.

Cook the rice according to the package directions.

Combine the cooked rice with the sour cream and season with salt. Spread half of the mixture in a buttered casserole dish. Top with the cubed cheese and the chopped chilies. Spread the remaining rice mixture over the top. Sprinkle with the grated cheese. Dot with butter. Bake, covered, for 30 minutes at 350° F.

This recipe can be prepared ahead of time and refrigerated or frozen, and then thawed for one hour and baked.

MAKES 10 SERVINGS

❧ HERBED ORANGE RICE

(Palos Presbyterian Church)

1 cup dry rice
⅔ cup chopped celery with leaves
2 tablespoons minced onion
4 tablespoons (½ stick) butter
1 cup water
1 cup orange juice
1 tablespoon grated orange zest
1 teaspoon salt
⅛ teaspoon thyme leaves

Cook the rice according to package directions.

While the rice is cooking, in a medium skillet, sauté the celery and onion in the butter for 5 to 10 minutes, until tender.

Add the remaining ingredients. Heat to boiling and then add to the cooked rice. Reduce the heat and simmer, covered, until the liquid is absorbed.

HINT: Crumble the orange zest before adding. It has a tendency to stick together.

MAKES 2–4 SERVINGS

❧ SPANISH RICE

3 slices bacon, diced
1 onion, diced
½ cup rice
1 14½-ounce can peeled tomatoes, chopped
Salt and pepper

Preheat the oven to 400°F.

In a medium skillet, cook the bacon and onion.

In a medium saucepan, make the rice according to the package directions, bringing it to a boil and simmering 45 minutes until well cooked. Add the bacon, onion, tomatoes, salt, and pepper and stir well. Pour into a casserole, cover, and bake 40 minutes in a 400°F. oven.

MAKES 2–4 SERVINGS

❧ SAUCE FOR BROCCOLI OR CAULIFLOWER
(Janet Bolser)

¼ cup LEGAL mayonnaise
¼ cup grated sharp cheddar cheese
1 to 2 pinches of dried minced onions

Mix the ingredients in a glass bowl and cook in the microwave on medium high until bubbly. Stir into the cooked hot vegetables before serving.

Try this as a dip for raw veggies.

⇜ MUSHROOM AND WILD RICE STUFFING

4 tablespoons (½ stick) unsalted butter
½ pound or 1 4-ounce can sliced mushrooms
¼ cup minced onion
1 tablespoon minced flat-leaf parsley
½ cup chopped celery
2 cups cooked wild rice
¾ teaspoon salt
Dash of pepper

In a large skillet, melt the butter until it sizzles. Add the mushrooms and sauce until tender, about 5 minutes. Remove the onions and set aside.

Add the onions, parsley, and celery to the skillet and cook until the onions are tender. Stir in the rice, salt, pepper, and the mushrooms.

This recipe makes enough stuffing for a 4- to 5-pound chicken. You can also make stuffing with dried prunes and/or apple slices.

⋘ ESCARGOTS

1 dozen canned snails with shells
4 tablespoons (½ stick) unsalted butter
1 teaspoon flat-leaf parsley, finely chopped
1 teaspoon minced garlic
1 teaspoon finely chopped shallot
1 teaspoon salt
⅛ teaspoon pepper
Dash of nutmeg

Preheat the oven to 350°F.

Drain the canned snails through a strainer. Clean the shells and place the snails in the shells. Place the snails and shells in a baking dish.

In a small skillet, melt the butter. Sauté the parsley, garlic, and shallot until tender. Add the salt, pepper, and nutmeg.

Pour the sauce over the snails and bake 20 minutes, or until the butter sauce just begins to boil.

MAKES 2 SERVINGS

❧ ROASTED PEPPER AND TOMATO SAUCE

(Luanne Greenberg)

2 tablespoons extra-virgin olive oil

1 large onion, chopped

1 7-ounce jar roasted red peppers, diced

2 garlic cloves, finely chopped

1 dried chili pepper

*12 fresh plum tomatoes, stemmed and chopped, or 1 28-
ounce can whole tomatoes, drained and coarsely
chopped*

1 teaspoon salt

½ teaspoon freshly ground black pepper

12 fresh basil leaves, chopped

Grated Parmesan or Romano cheese (optional)

Heat the oil in a medium skillet over medium-high heat. Add
the onion; cook until softened, about 2 minutes. Add the red
peppers, garlic, chili pepper, and tomatoes; cook, uncovered,
until bubbling vigorously, about 4 minutes. Stir in the salt, pepper, and basil; cook 1 minute. Remove the chili pepper. Serve
over chicken, and sprinkle with cheese if desired.

Luanne likes to make this sauce, pour it over boneless
chicken, and then top with freshly grated Parmesan
(canned Parmesan has dextrose to prevent clumping).
She serves a salad and rice to accompany the chicken.
It has become one of her family's favorites.

MAKES 6–8 SERVINGS

⤳ BÉARNAISE SAUCE

3 tablespoons vinegar

1 teaspoon finely chopped green onion or shallot

4 peppercorns, crushed

1 bouquet garni of a few tarragon and chervil leaves

4 egg yolks

8 tablespoons (1 stick) unsalted butter, at room temperature

Salt to taste

1 teaspoon fresh tarragon or ¼ teaspoon dried tarragon

In a small saucepan, combine the vinegar, green onion, peppercorn, and bouquet garni. Simmer until the liquid is reduced by half. Strain into a small bowl. Add 1 tablespoon of cold water to the herb liquid.

Off the heat, beat the egg yolks in the top of a double boiler. Slowly add the herb liquid. Have the butter ready at room temperature.

Add a few tablespoons of the butter to the egg-yolk mixture. Place in the double boiler over hot, but not boiling, water. Cook and stir until the butter melts and the sauce starts to thicken. Continue adding butter until the consistency is that of a smooth cream.

Add salt and tarragon and serve.

❧ HONEY DIJON DRESSING

(Lailah Leeser)

6 to 7 ounces brown spicy mustard
2 tablespoons honey
2 tablespoons vinegar
Poppy seeds

In a medium bowl, whisk together all the ingredients. Serve.

❧ BLUE CHEESE SALAD DRESSING

(Mike Yeager)

1 pint sour cream
4 to 6 ounces blue cheese, softened

Using a hand mixer, blend the ingredients together. Refrigerate overnight to improve the flavor. The dressing will keep for 2 to 3 weeks.

❧ SLUSH

(Judith Kuncel)

8 ounces sour cream
1 12-ounce package frozen fruit, slightly defrosted
1 teaspoon vanilla
Honey or Equal to taste

Mix all of the ingredients in a blender. Freeze in a sealable freezer container and scoop out servings as needed.

☙ HONEY BARBECUE BASTE

(Luanne Greenberg)

1 tablespoon vegetable oil
¼ cup minced onion
1 garlic clove, minced
1 8-ounce can tomato sauce
1 6-ounce can tomato paste
⅓ cup honey
3 tablespoons vinegar
1 teaspoon dry mustard
½ teaspoon salt
¼ teaspoon coarsely ground black pepper

Heat the oil in a medium saucepan over medium heat until hot. Add the onion and garlic; cook and stir until the onion is tender. Add the remaining ingredients. Bring to a boil; reduce heat to low and simmer 20 minutes. Serve over grilled chicken, pork, spareribs, salmon, or hamburgers.

☙ KNOX BLOX

(Dar)

4 envelopes Knox unflavored gelatin
3 3-ounce packages flavored sugar-free gelatin
4 cups boiling water

In a large bowl, combine the unflavored and flavored gelatin; add the boiling water and stir until the gelatin is completely dissolved. Pour into a 9 × 13-inch pan and chill until firm. Cut into squares to serve.

MAKES 100 ONE-INCH SQUARES

❧ CINNAMON APPLES

(Mary Paul)

Cut apples into slices. Put in a plastic bag with cinnamon and Equal to taste. Shake and put in the refrigerator. Eat when cold.

This is a great snack food.

❧ THREE-BERRY SHAKE

(Luanne Greenberg)

> *1 pint fresh strawberries, hulled and halved*
> *½ cup skim milk*
> *¼ cup fresh blueberries*
> *¼ cup fresh raspberries*
> *½ small ripe banana, sliced*
> *Equal, to taste*
> *1 cup ice cubes*
> *Mint sprigs, for garnish*

Combine the strawberries, milk, blueberries, raspberries, banana, Equal, and ice cubes in a blender; puree until smooth. Garnish with mint.

MAKES 2 SERVINGS

⤳ GRANOLA

(Victoria Adamson)

4 cups Quaker Quick oats
1 cup nuts and seeds (chopped if large)
2 teaspoons cinnamon
2 tablespoons vanilla
6 ounces apple juice concentrate (½ can of frozen concentrate)
1½ cups minced dried fruit (raisins, apricots, peaches, cranberries, blueberries)
Cream
Equal

Nothing is going to go wrong with this recipe if the amounts are changed. Feel free to add and subtract ingredients as your taste dictates.

⤳ TABBOULEH

(Terrie Gray)

12 ounces bulgur (cracked wheat)
1 large bunch of flat-leaf parsley, chopped
1 medium onion, chopped
2 to 3 pounds tomatoes, chopped
¾ cup freshly squeezed lemon juice
¾ cup olive oil
Salt and pepper

Wrap the bulgur in a tea towel, run water over it to wash it, and squeeze out the excess water. Place in a large bowl. Mix in the remaining ingredients and stir well. Let stand in the refrigerator at least 2 hours and preferably overnight to blend the flavors.

MAYONNAISE

> *1 egg yolk*
> *1 teaspoon dry mustard*
> *1 teaspoon honey*
> *¼ teaspoon salt*
> *Dash of cayenne pepper*
> *2 tablespoons lemon juice or vinegar*
> *1 cup vegetable oil*

In a medium bowl with an electric beater, beat together the egg yolk, mustard, honey, salt, cayenne pepper, and 1 tablespoon of the lemon juice. Continue beating while adding the vegetable oil, at first drop by drop, gradually increasing the amount as the mixture thickens until all of the oil has been added. Slowly add the last tablespoon of lemon juice. Beat well. Chill.

MAKES 1½ CUPS OF MAYONNAISE

GUACAMOLE

> *2 avocados, peeled*
> *1 tablespoon grated onion*
> *1 tablespoon freshly squeezed lemon juice*
> *1 teaspoon salt*
> *¼ teaspoon chili powder*
> *⅓ cup mayonnaise*

In a medium glass bowl, mash the avocados with a fork. Stir in the onion, lemon juice, salt, and chili powder.

Spread the mayonnaise over the mixture, sealing it to the edges of the bowl. Chill. At serving time, blend in the mayonnaise. Serve with fresh-cut vegetables.

◈ MEXICAN CEVICHE (SOUTH TEXAS STYLE)

(Ed Moreno)

1 pound uncooked flounder or red snapper, chopped fine
2 to 3 canned pickled jalapeños, chopped fine, juice
  reserved
Freshly squeezed juice of 10 to 15 key limes
Salt
2 medium tomatoes, diced
1 medium onion, chopped fine
1 cup cilantro, chopped fine

In a plastic bowl with a lid, combine the fish, pickled jalapeño juice, and lime juice and mix well. Add a pinch of salt, tomatoes, onion, jalapeños, and cilantro and mix well. Cover and refrigerate overnight.

MAKES 4–6 SERVINGS

DESSERTS

DR. DOROTHY'S SWEET TREATS
(Cleo Ullom)

Honey
1 cup crushed Shredded Wheat (don't break too fine)
½ cup Grape-Nuts
½ cup plump raisins
½ cup dried papayas, chopped (not dried with sugar)
1 cup lightly toasted pecan halves or pieces
Salt to taste (optional)
1 cup finely chopped pecans

In a medium bowl, warm a small amount of honey in a microwave. Stir in all the remaining ingredients except the chopped pecans. Butter hands and make the mixture into small balls. Be careful to use just enough honey to hold the mixture together—otherwise the balls will remain sticky. Roll balls in the chopped pecans.

MAKES 1 DOZEN

NO-BAKE CHEESECAKE
(Susan Sphar)

1 envelope Knox gelatin
1 cup cold water
2 8-ounce packages cream cheese, softened
12 packages Equal
1 teaspoon vanilla
Fresh fruit, sliced (optional)

In a small saucepan, sprinkle the gelatin over ¼ cup of the cold water; let stand 1 minute. Stir over low heat until the gelatin is completely dissolved.

In a large bowl, with an electric mixer, beat the cream cheese, Equal, and vanilla until blended. Gradually beat in the gelatin mixture and the remaining ¾ cup water until smooth. Pour into a pie plate. Chill until firm. Garnish, if desired, with fresh fruit.

MAKES 6–8 SERVINGS

❧ HONEY VANILLA ICE CREAM
(Elizabeth Holt)

6 large eggs
1 quart milk
1 cup honey
1 quart whipping cream
2 tablespoons vanilla extract

Combine the eggs, milk, and honey in a large saucepan. Cook over low heat, stirring constantly, 20 to 25 minutes, or until the mixture thickens and coats a spoon. Cool and then stir in the whipping cream and vanilla. Cover and chill at least 8 hours.

Pour the mixture into a 5-quart, hand-turned or electric ice-cream freezer. Freeze according to manufacturer's instructions.

> This is to be eaten *after* you've lost weight, and then only for special occasions. Also, you must share. You are not allowed to eat the whole gallon by yourself at one or even two sittings!

MAKES 1 GALLON

⤳ MACAROONS

(Susan Sphar)

1 cup honey
½ cup milk
½ teaspoon baking soda
1 teaspoon vanilla
3 to 3½ cups rolled oats
6 tablespoons unsweetened cocoa
1 cup chopped nuts
1 cup shredded unsweetened coconut

In a large saucepan, cook the honey, milk, and baking soda over medium heat until the temperature reaches 250°F. on a candy thermometer. Do not scorch the mixture by having the heat too high.

When the honey mixture has reached 250°F., remove it from the heat and add the vanilla. Next, add the oats, cocoa, nuts, and coconut. Mix quickly, then drop by teaspoonsful onto waxed paper. You may also press the mixture onto a cookie sheet and cut it into squares when cool.

> HINT: Susan says they're *great* when eaten with fresh strawberries and a spoonful of homemade whipped cream on top. (And you are not allowed to eat more than one a day of these—*after* you've lost the weight.)

MAKES 2–3 DOZEN

✑ SORBET

For this recipe I like to use frozen strawberries, raspberries, mangos, blackberries, and anything else I can find that hasn't had sugar added.

Partially defrost the fruit. Put some of each into a blender. Add a banana and Equal to taste and almost cover with half and half. Blend well. Pour into sherbet glasses for guests or into disposable aluminum cupcake cups for yourself. Cover with foil and place in the freezer.

> This sorbet is a great treat, especially during the summer.

✑ EGG CUSTARD

(Nancy Nance)
3 eggs, slightly beaten
¼ teaspoon salt
¼ cup honey or Equal
2 cups scalded milk, cooled
½ teaspoon vanilla
Nutmeg (optional)

In a Crock-Pot, combine the eggs, salt, and honey. Slowly stir in the cooled milk and the vanilla. Add nutmeg to taste. Cook on low until a knife inserted off-center comes out clean, 3 to 4 hours.

MAKES 4 SERVINGS

MISCELLANEOUS

"SOUTH OF THE BORDER"— SAUCE FOR STEAK

(Santa Teresa Country Club, Santa Teresa, New Mexico)

2 onions, chopped
½ pound long green chile peppers, pre-cooked
½ pound tomatoes, fresh or canned, diced
Salt and pepper to taste
1 pound white cheddar cheese, melted
1 pint of heavy cream

Sauté the onions and chile peppers. Stir in the tomatoes and salt and pepper. Add the melted cheese and cream, mixing until well-blended.

MAKES 1 GALLON

PIZZA CRUST

(Cleo Ullom)

1 cup crushed Shredded Wheat
1 egg white, beaten stiff
Olive oil

Preheat the oven to 275°F.

In a medium bowl, combine the Shredded Wheat and the egg whites. Spread evenly in the bottom and up the sides of a 13-inch pizza pan or other baking pan. Bake for 30 to 60 minutes, or until firm.

Remove the crust from the oven and spread it with a touch of olive oil to keep tomatoes from soaking into the crust. Add your favorite LEGAL toppings.

⌘ OATMEAL APPLE CINNAMON MUFFINS

(Annalee Johnson)

½ cup Grape-Nuts
¾ cup rolled oats
½ teaspoon salt
2 tablespoons melted unsalted butter
1 beaten egg
½ teaspoon cinnamon
⅓ cup honey
1 small apple, grated
¼ cup unsweetened applesauce (or ½ cup applesauce
    without the grated apple)

Preheat the oven to 425°F.

Spray a muffin tin with cooking spray, or line the tin with paper liners.

Mix all the ingredients together. Spoon into the muffin tin and bake for 20 minutes, or until a toothpick comes out with just a few crumbs.

MAKES 6–12 SERVINGS

⤇ APPLESAUCE

⅓ teaspoon cinnamon
14 apples, washed, peeled, cored, and cut into chunks
2 tablespoons Equal, or to taste

In a large saucepan, toss the cinnamon with the apples. Add a small amount of water and bring to a boil; reduce the heat and simmer until tender.

Remove the applesauce from the heat and stir in the Equal.

CHAPTER 7

BITS AND PIECES

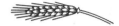

When fat is metabolized (broken down), it releases several substances plus carbon dioxide (which we breathe out) and water (which we urinate). When you urinate a lot, it isn't just all that water you are drinking; it is also the fat that is breaking down. So, be glad when you urinate a lot—you're losing weight!

To help you understand the importance of all that water, put yourself back into the chemistry lab. You have two beakers of powder, one with red powder and one with blue. You mix them together and nothing happens. Then you add water and the combined powders explode. The water was needed for the chemistry to happen. It is like that with our bodies. Even when we eat all of the right food, the breakdown of the fat doesn't happen as well without the water added to the equation.

For those of you who are having trouble getting all of your water in: *drink* your water, don't *sip* it. Also, pour your water into a glass or porcelain cup instead of plastic. The water tastes better in glass or porcelain. Another trick to get all of the water is to have a glass of water every time you go to the bathroom. You are going to wash your hands anyway, so you might as well have some water to drink while you are at the sink.

When you go to the grocery store, you should be spending most of your time in the outside aisles. The outside aisles usually have the fresh fruits and vegetables; the meat, fish, and fowl; and the dairy products. The more time you spend in those inner aisles, the more likely you are to get contaminated and illegal food.

Don't have cereal more than once a day. Don't do it. It will slow you down. Remember, a variety of food every day is the key.

As far as eating *anything* in unlimited amounts goes, only veggies fit in that category. Even so, eating only veggies and not fruits, protein, or fat is not following God's Diet. You shouldn't be a glutton with any food.

I have not talked about amounts of each food or each meal because there are not very many of us who have the exact same age, same sex, same build, same metabolism, same work, and same expenditure of calories. If you aren't losing weight, look at the quantity of each food you are eating. If you are heavier on the fruits than the veggies, switch it. Don't forget to have protein every day. Are you still drinking a half gallon of coffee or tea every day? Get rid of it!

Beware of nuts. Many have had cornstarch added to them. Be sure to read the ingredients on the label. Also, nuts should be limited to a maximum of a handful each day. If you are finding that you are eating too many, either don't buy them or buy them in the shell. After all, shelled is the way God made them and it will slow down your consumption of them when you have to work for the treat.

Catherine Dorman shares a neat idea. Get those adhesive dot stickers in red and green. When you go through your pantry after reading this book to see what you should and shouldn't eat, label all of the cans and packages that are illegal with red dots and put the green dots on the good food.

One of my patients suggests that when we are offered something "illegal" we say: "Sorry. I DON'T eat that," rather than the usual "I CAN'T eat that." (The mind-set can make a difference. After all, we CAN eat anything we want. We simply don't choose to eat something illegal because we know better than that.)

LEGAL foods: Cardini makes some salad dressings that are sugar-free. Look at the labels carefully, since they also make some "contaminated" ones. You can find these at most grocery stores.

There are a few typically illegal foods that the manufacturer has made "legally."

Un-ketchup
Annie's Ranch Dressing
Hain Mayonnaise with safflower or canola
Daisy Sour Cream
Price's 4% Cottage Cheese
Horizon Vanilla Yogurt

Check your grocery shelves for others. Many of our packaged foods are distributed locally, so what I have available may not be in your area, and vice versa.

Equal has produced several recipe books that you can get for free. They have an 800 number on their packaging. While they still have some contaminated recipes, they also have many that are legal. Call them for your free copies of the recipe books to get some extra ideas for cooking. Do not heat Equal, as it becomes bitter.

Several of our elite group of enlightened patients have shared with me how to thicken gravies. I pass their ideas on to you to try: Stir in sour cream, buttermilk, or crumbled hard-boiled egg yolk. Cook until thickened.

If someone says that your cholesterol and triglycerides will go up, they are wrong. I've got the statistics to prove that these test values, as well as elevated blood sugar levels (and even insulin dosages for diabetics), go down.

Beware of *any* canned or packaged food. Read the *ingredients,* not the percent or grams of calories, fat, protein, and carbohydrates. Our enemies are SUGAR, FLOUR, CORN SYRUP, and CORNSTARCH.

Beware of anything that says "low fat" or "all natural." Those are often the worst for added sugar, corn syrup, or cornstarch.

❦

Fried foods are not good—so try to avoid them.

❦

Just as you shouldn't overdo on the nuts, so you shouldn't overdo with dried fruit or fruit juices. They will slow you down. If you wouldn't have ten fresh oranges a day, so you shouldn't have ten oranges' worth of orange juice a day. You wouldn't eat fifteen fresh apricots, so don't eat that much in dried apricots, either.

Limit your caffeine (coffee, tea, and sodas) to a total of two cups or glasses per day. Best would be none at all. The caffeine stimulates the pancreas to produce insulin, which then takes the glucose out of our blood and puts it on our hips. Caffeine also acts as a mild diuretic, which then depletes us of the water we need to help break down the fat. Caffeine can cause mild dehydration, leading to fatigue. Caffeine is a drug and really should be on the list of never to have. I've never gone through withdrawal when I stopped broccoli or chicken, but I've sure gone through withdrawal when I stopped caffeine!

Honey is precious. Eat it that way. Remember our caveman who knocked down the beehive and risked death? If you had to risk death for honey as he did, you *would* treat it as something *very precious.*

Sugar, flour, corn syrup, and cornstarch are DRUGS. They are addictive and when you eliminate them from your diet, you will go through withdrawal. Treat them with the respect you would give drugs and stay away from them.

CHAPTER 8

CONCLUSION

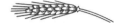

IF GOD DIDN'T MAKE IT, DON'T EAT IT.

When you read the lists of foods, make sure that you check everything that is packaged. For example, not all sour cream is good and not all soy sauce is bad. Read the ingredients. Your enemies are SUGAR, FLOUR, CORN SYRUP, and CORN-STARCH.

This way of eating is a way of life. Make food your friend and not your enemy.

Drink 8 to 10 of the 8-ounce glasses of water a day.

Walk half an hour every day.

Enjoy life.

NOTES

❧

1. Ginger Thompson, "Adult-type Diabetes Develops Among Teens," *The New York Times,* 14 December 1998.

2. Kalpana Srinivasan, "Government Coalition Formulates Diet Industry Guidelines," *El Paso Times* (Texas), 10 February 1999.

3. Lori Johntson, "Obesity, Smoking Linked to Type of Esophagus Cancer," *El Paso Times* (Texas), 13 November 1998.

4. C. Wayne Callaway, M.D., referencing work done by H.N. Ginsberg, W. Karmally, M. Siddiqui et al., in "A Special Report," *Post-Graduate Medicine,* June 1997.

5. Kathryn M. Rexrode, M.D., and Brigham and Women's Hospital, Boston, "Obesity, Weight Gain Boost Stroke in Women," *Journal of the American Medical Association* (1997) 277:1539–45.

6. J. Carper, "Table Sugar May Shorten Life Span, Increase Aging," *El Paso Times* (Texas), 25 September 1995.

7. National Task Force on the Prevention and Treatment of Obesity, "Long-term Pharmacotherapy in the Management of Obesity," *Journal of the American Medical Association* (1996) 276:1907–15.

8. "School Menus," *El Paso Times* (Texas), 7 March 1999, 6B.

9. Jennifer Read Holman, "Foods that Boost Your Moods," *Reader's Digest,* February 1996 (condensed from original in *Ladies Home Journal*).

10. *Taber's Cyclopedic Medical Dictionary.* Philadelphia: F.A. Davis Company, 1986.

11. Robert A. Atkins, M.D. *Dr. Atkins' Diet Revolution.* New York: David McKay, 1972.

12. *Merriam Webster's Collegiate Dictionary.* Springfield, Mass.: Merriam Webster, Inc., 1996.

13. *The Merck Manual.* Rahway, N.J.: Merck Sharpe & Dohme Research Laboratories, 1987.

INDEX

❧

CONVERSION CHART
EQUIVALENT IMPERIAL AND METRIC MEASUREMENTS

American cooks use standard containers, the 8-ounce cup and a tablespoon that takes exactly 16 level fillings to fill that cup level. Measuring by cup makes it very difficult to give weight equivalents, as a cup of densely packed butter will weigh considerably more than a cup of flour. The easiest way therefore to deal with cup measurements in recipes is to take the amount by volume rather than by weight. Thus the equation reads:

1 cup = 240 ml = 8 fl. oz.
½ cup = 120 ml = 4 fl. oz.

It is possible to buy a set of American cup measures in major stores around the world.

In the States, butter is often measured in sticks. One stick is the equivalent of 8 tablespoons. One tablespoon of butter is therefore the equivalent to ½ ounce/15 grams.

LIQUID MEASURES

Fluid Ounces	U.S.	Imperial	Milliliters
	1 tsp	1 tsp	5
¼	2 tsps	1 dessert-spoon	10
½	1 tb	1 tbn	14
1	2 tbs	2 tbs	28
2	¼ cup	4 tbs	56
4	½ cup		110
5		¼ pt or 1 gill	140
6	¾ cup		170
8	1 cup		225
9			250, ¼ liter
10	1¼ cups	½ pt	280
12	1½ cups		340
15		¾ pt	420
16	2 cups		450
18	2¼ cups		500, ½ liter
20	2½ cups	1 pt	560
24	3 cups or 1½ pts		675
25		1¼ pts	700
27	3½ cups		750, ¾ liter
30	3¾ cups	1½ pts	840
32	4 cups or 2 pts or 1 qt		900
35		1¾ pts	980
36	4½ cups		1000, 1 liter
40	5 cups	2 pts or 1 qt	1120

SOLID MEASURES

U.S. and Imperial		Metric	
Ounces	Pounds	Grams	Kilos
1		28	
2		56	
3½		100	
4	¼	112	
5		140	
6		168	
8	½	225	
9		250	¼
12	¾	340	
16	1	450	

OVEN TEMPERATURE EQUIVALENTS

F	C	Gas Mark	Description
225	110	¼	Cool
250	130	½	
275	140	1	Very Slow
300	150	2	
325	170	3	Slow
350	180	4	Moderate
375	190	5	
400	200	6	Moderately Hot
425	220	7	Fairly Hot
450	230	8	Hot
475	240	9	Very Hot
500	250	10	Extremely Hot

Any broiling recipes can be used with the grill of the oven, but beware of high-temperature grills.

EQUIVALENTS FOR INGREDIENTS

all-purpose flour—plain flour
arugula—rocket
beet—beetroot
coarse salt—kitchen salt
cornstarch—cornflour
eggplant—aubergine
fava beans—broad beans
granulated sugar—caster sugar
lima beans—broad beans
scallion—spring onion
shortening—white fat
snow pea—mangetout
squash—courgettes or marrow
unbleached flour—strong, white flour
zest—rind
zucchini—courgettes or marrow
baking sheet—oven tray
plastic wrap—cling film

ABOUT THE AUTHOR

❧

Dr. Dorothy Gault-McNemee, M.D., called "Dr. Dorothy" by friends, colleagues, and patients, was born and raised in Chicago, Illinois. After graduating from Roosevelt University, she earned her doctor of medicine at the Autonomous University of Guadalajara. She completed a rotating internship at Cook County Hospital in Chicago and an internship in pediatrics at Texas Tech University Health Sciences Center.

Dr. Dorothy built the Doctors of Santa Teresa Medical Clinic in Santa Teresa, New Mexico, where she employs three full-time physicians, one part-time physician, and a staff of twenty-two employees. Prior to establishing Doctors of Santa Teresa, she designed and built Santa Teresa Immediate Care Center for Hotel Dieu Hospital. She is a member of the American Board of Certification in Family Practice and is certified as a Medical Review Officer and an FAA Medical Examiner.

God's Diet, a no-nonsense and practical method of maintaining a healthy eating style, was a self-published, regional best-seller.

Contact Dr. Dorothy at the Doctors of Santa Teresa Medical Clinic Web site at www.doctorsofsantateresa.com, or e-mail her at drst@doctorsofsantateresa.com.